BALANCE HORMONES NATURALLY

by

Kate Neil and Patrick Holford

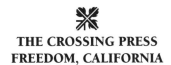

THE CROSSING PRESS
FREEDOM, CALIFORNIA

Acknowledgments

This book would not have been possible without the help of many people. Our thanks go to Dr John Lee, Martin Neil, Jan Shepheard, Natalie Savona and the team at Piatkus for their guidance and support.

Copyright © 1999 by Kate Neil and Patrick Holford
Published by The Crossing Press in 1999
First published in the U.K. by Judy Piatkus (Publishers) Ltd in 1998
Printed in the U.S.A.
Cover design by Victoria May
Interior illustration by Jonathan Phillips and Christopher Quayle

For information on bulk purchases or group discounts for this and other Crossing Press titles, please contact our Special Sales Manager at (800) 777-1048. Visit our Web site: **www.crossingpress.com**

Library of Congress Cataloging-in-Publication Data

Neil, Kate.
 Balance hormones naturally / by Kate Neil and Patrick Holford.
     p. cm.
 Includes bibliographical references and index.
 ISBN 0-58091-041-6 (pbk.)
     1. Women--Diseases Popular works. 2. Women--Diseases--Nutritional
aspects. 3. Women--Nutrition. 4. Women--Dieseases --diet therapy.
I. Holford, Patrick. II. Title.
  RG121.N44   1999
    618.'.04654--dc21
                                                    98-33919
                                                       CIP

CONTENTS

INTRODUCTION

For the first time since the introduction of the contraceptive pill, and the subsequent massive rise in synthetic hormone use, there are proven natural alternatives available to help prevent and treat most female health problems.

It is only now, 40 years on, that the real long-term effects of taking synthetic hormones are being fully realized. Even though some medical researchers back in the 1960s were well aware of the potential side-effects of taking synthetic hormones, those with the power to make final decisions considered that the benefits far outweighed any risks.

Without any doubt, pharmaceutical companies had a lot to gain financially from the widespread prescription of synthetic hormones. Women of all ages were potential customers. Sex hormones not only act as contraceptives, but are also widely used in infertility programs, and are regularly recommended in the form of Hormone Replacement Therapy (HRT) to keep the menopause at bay. With the accepted use of synthetic hormones as reliable contraceptives, research into natural estrogens and progesterone declined rapidly, as high profits could not be made from the sale of natural, unpatentable products.

For sex hormones – natural or synthetic – to be optimally effective it is crucial that they are in balance. Today it is very hard for our bodies, even under the best of circumstances, to keep our sex hormones balanced. So what is happening to women? We are currently living in a sea of estrogenic compounds which are found in food, air and water, plastic residues, exhaust fumes and pesticides. We eat, drink and breathe them into our bodies.

THE NEW PROBLEM OF ESTROGEN DOMINANCE

Many current female health problems are linked to having too much estrogen in the body. These include PMS, endometriosis, ovarian cysts, fibroids, breast cancer and menopausal problems. Dr John Lee from Sebastopol, California, has defined a new syndrome, "Estrogen Dominance," to explain many of these common female conditions. Dr Lee has had two decades of clinical experience in the field of female health, and his published research explains clearly the background to his theory that many women are suffering from the effects of too much estrogen. He believes that stress, nutritional deficiencies, estrogenic substances from the environment, and taking synthetic estrogens, combined with a deficiency of progesterone, are all likely contributory factors in the creation of estrogen dominance.

THE ROLE OF WOMEN

Women play a very powerful, indeed pivotal, role in society, of which they are largely unaware. The responsibility of nourishing themselves and the family has traditionally always been left to them but it is only in this last decade that the importance of nutrition has been realized. So much so, that the future health and survival of the whole human race depends very much upon sound nutrition. Largely due to the dominance of men in medicine, and the subordinate role most women have historically played in society, women's understanding and acceptance of themselves has been greatly influenced by the ideas of men. We believe that most women have an inherent knowledge of their own natural way of being, and are happiest when they are free to live according to it.

It is time for women to become educated and clear about what is happening to their own bodies, to take responsibility for their health, and to live a life that is in harmony with their natural design.

It is our experience, in both teaching and advising women about hormones, that their overall understanding is very sketchy. They are usually amazed at the marvelous synchrony that regulates the peaks and troughs of the monthly cycle for around 40 years of their life.

Making simple and beneficial changes to your diet and lifestyle are the first important steps towards balanced hormones and better health. To help you along the way, natural hormonal preparations are now available. When combined with adjustments in diet and lifestyle, these can help restore the natural hormone balance in your body and return you to a state of good, natural health.

Guide to Abbreviations and Measures

1 gram (g) = 1000 milligrams (mg) = 1,000,000 micrograms (mcg or µg).

Most vitamins are measured in milligrams or micrograms. Vitamins A, D and E are also measured in International Units (iu), a measurement designed to standardize the different forms of these vitamins that have different potencies.

1 mcg of retinol (mcg RE) = 3.3iu of vitamin A

1mcg RE of beta-carotene = 6mcg of beta-carotene

100iu of vitamin D = 2.5mcg

100iu of vitamin E = 67mg

1 pound (lb) = 16 ounces (oz)   2.2 lb = 1 kilogram (kg)

1 pint = 0.6 litres   1.76 pints = 1 litre

In this book calories means kilocalories (kcal)

PART 1

UNDERSTANDING YOUR BODY

CHAPTER 1

THE FEMALE LIFE CYCLE

Women are meant to be in harmony with their bodies – they have developed a natural monthly rhythm in which hormone levels ebb and flow. This is as nature planned, and provided your diet, environment and lifestyle conform to your natural design, then no part of the female life cycle need be thought of as an illness or a disabling condition.

There are three main hormonal phases in a woman's life: menstruation, pregnancy and menopause. Understanding each of these helps you take control and make clear decisions about what you need.

The sex hormones, progesterone and estrogens, play a key role in all stages of the female health cycle. Knowing how they work and what they do is vital for any woman who wants to be sure of her hormonal health.

Until relatively recently, the bodies of men and women were considered structurally similar. In the fourth century the Bishop of Emesa in Syria wrote, "Women have the same genitalia as men except that theirs are inside the body and not outside it." It was not until 1890 that medical science began to investigate the workings of the human menstrual cycle.

As medicine was, and still is, largely dominated by men, the current understanding of the female cycle and female problems is based on a male perspective. The language that medical and scientific men once used to describe the processes that occur throughout the female life cycle still colours our understanding and attitudes today.

In previous centuries it was extremely rare to find accounts of women's views on what they thought was happening to their bodies. Women have thereby come to understand the workings of their bodies through men. However, by the 1950s, women started to question what was happening to them; and, as a result, the natural childbirth and women's rights movements began to develop.

Attempts to control fertility must be as old as childbirth itself. What is new, in the second half of this century, is the method of control. For the first time in human history, drugs have been widely used for the purpose of birth control. Although it was known that these drugs would control fertility, the full implications of their effects on health were not fully realized. It is only now that we are beginning to have a good understanding, not only of the effects of these drugs, but of the intricate synchrony of events that control the monthly cycle.

NATURE'S DESIGN

The female pelvis is truly a wonder to behold. It contains the uterus which, under the influence of a fine balance of hormones, prepares for itself every month a special lining in case of pregnancy. If pregnancy does not occur, this lining is shed and the process of building up a new one starts again. The uterus is normally smaller than a fist but can accommodate a baby larger than a football. It contains muscles like no others found in the body: through regular uterine contraction and retraction they can successfully deliver a baby and yet return to normal size within only six weeks. The ovaries are responsible for producing eggs and are enclosed in sacs that are well protected, deep within the pelvic cavity. Nature finds very ingenious ways of ensuring the survival of the species.

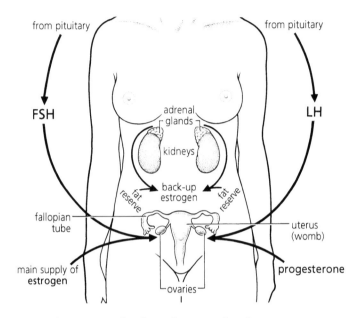

from pituitary

from pituitary

FSH

LH

adrenal glands

kidneys

back-up estrogen

fat reserve

fat reserve

fallopian tube

uterus (womb)

main supply of estrogen

progesterone

ovaries

Figure 1 – The female reproductive system

THE FEMALE LIFE CYCLE

The sex hormones in girls remain dormant until about the age of 11 to 13. Around then, the hypothalamus, a small gland at the base of the brain, makes a master hormone. This instructs the pituitary gland connected to it to release into the blood two powerful hormones, follicle stimulating hormone (FSH) and luteinizing hormone (LH). These two hormones are responsible for the development and release of an egg from the ovary. When a girl is approaching the onset of her menstrual cycle, the cells of the pituitary gland and ovary are laden with receptors, which become super-sensitive to these stimulating hormones. It takes about three years for the menstrual cycle to become fully established from the time of the first period. Of the millions of potentially mature eggs that are present before birth, only about 300,000 are left at puberty.

The Menstrual Cycle

It is worth remembering that the only purpose of the monthly menstrual cycle is to ensure the survival of the species. In regular, precisely synchronized order, the sex hormones are released into the blood to bring about the release of a mature healthy egg, in the hope that it will meet an equally healthy sperm and become fertilized by it. The cycle repeats itself, month after month, for around 40 years of a woman's life, and is normally interrupted only by pregnancy.

The master of this hormonal activity is the hypothalamus. It acts like a control center which shares and integrates many biochemical, immunological and emotional conditions. Menstruation can be affected by emotional states, stress, diet, other hormones, illness and drugs. The average menstrual cycle lasts for 28 days, although it is not uncommon for cycles to vary between three to six weeks.

From Menstruation to Ovulation (Days 1–14)

At the beginning of a menstrual cycle the levels of the hormones estrogen and progesterone are very low as a result of the shedding of the specially prepared uterine lining. This happens when a fully mature egg is not fertilized by a sperm.

The hypothalamus gland senses that the levels of estrogen and progesterone are low and releases the first master hormone which causes the pituitary gland to release follicle stimulating hormone (FSH). As the name implies, FSH works on the eggs within the ovary, ripening one for release and fertilisation. FSH also stimulates the production of estrogen by the ovary; levels of this gradually rise over the first half of the cycle, bringing about the growth of the lining of the uterus and breast tissue. This process lasts about ten days and is sometimes known as the proliferative stage of the cycle. It sets the scene for the reception of a fertilized egg.

Follicles are ripened and prepared in both ovaries.

Estrogen levels peak around day 12 of the cycle, which gives a signal to the hypothalamus gland to release luteinizing hormone (LH). On day 14 of a normal cycle, a surge of LH brings about ovulation, the release of a mature egg from one of the ovaries. The egg is now free to enter and move down the fallopian tube attached to the uterus. Helped by specialized hair-like tissue, the egg passes down the tube to meet the sperm.

From Ovulation to Menstruation (Days 14–28)

The space that is left behind in the ovary after the egg has been released fills with blood and specialized cells and builds up into a dense mass known as the corpus luteum. The corpus luteum now becomes the manufacturing site for both estrogens and progesterone during the second half of the cycle. High levels of both hormones are required to support fertilisation should it occur.

The rise of progesterone just after ovulation increases body temperature by at least $0.2°$ centigrade. Many women therefore take their temperature in order to check whether they have ovulated.

If the egg is not fertilized, the corpus luteum breaks down. The blood vessels supplying the uterine lining go into spasm and the lining is shed, forming the menstrual flow. The loss of the corpus luteum causes a rapid fall in the levels of estrogens and progesterone. This low level of estrogens and progesterone acts as a signal to the hypothalamus gland to release its master hormone and the process starts all over again (see Fig. 2 on page 7).

Pregnancy

If the egg does get fertilized, the corpus luteum continues to produce estrogens and progesterone in large quantities for the next 12 to 14 weeks, and in small quantities throughout

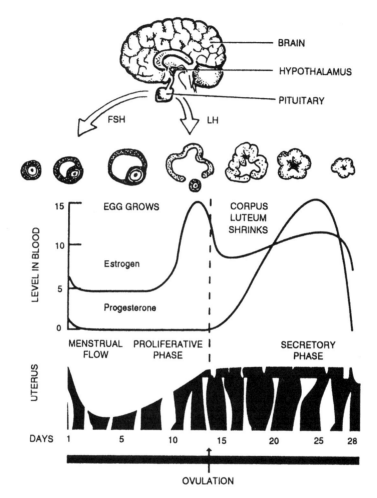

Figure 2 – Normal menstrual cycle

pregnancy. Once the fertilized egg has become embedded in the uterus, special cells made by the egg produce another hormone called human chorionic gonadotrophin (hCG).

This hormone stimulates the corpus luteum to continue growing for the next 12 to 14 weeks. By this time, the placenta is sufficiently developed to take over the production of both estrogens and progesterone to support the rest of the pregnancy. As levels of estrogens and progesterone are so high during pregnancy, the brain does not receive any messages from the egg-stimulating hormone FSH, or the ovulation hormone LH. Estrogen and progesterone levels do not fall again until the baby is due to be born.

Hormonal signals, about nine months after the first day of the last period, bring about labour (see Fig. 3 below).

Towards the time of labour, the womb becomes increasingly sensitive to oxytocin, a hormone whose action is stimulated by the pituitary gland. Oxytocin stimulates the uterus to contract, and begins and maintains the process of the delivery

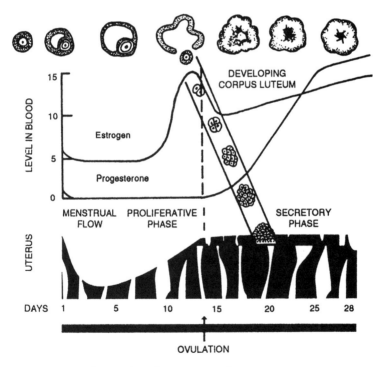

Figure 3 – First stage of pregnancy

of the baby. Contractions increase under the influence of oxytocin until the baby is born.

After delivery, levels of oestrogen and progesterone fall rapidly. Oestrogen remains low, and there is no rise in progesterone while a new mother is breastfeeding. Progesterone is not produced in any significant amount, as the mother is not ovulating. Breastfeeding is known to be a natural contraceptive, but, as the months of feeding pass or if the baby is receiving other kinds of food or supplements, it becomes an unreliable form of birth control.

Menopause

The menopause is a process that usually takes about ten years to complete and includes the period now commonly referred to as the "perimenopause" which is the five years or so before periods cease. Significant hormonal fluctuations continue during the first five years after the last period. It is the five years before and after the last period that is described as the menopause. The ovaries stop producing eggs and making oestrogens and progesterone. This process normally starts around the age of 45 and is usually complete by 55.

At the menopause, lower levels of estrogens are made because they are no longer needed to prepare the uterine lining for pregnancy. As estrogen levels fall, the menstrual flow becomes lighter and often quite irregular, until eventually it stops altogether. As the menopause progresses, many cycles occur in which an egg is not released. These are known as anovulatory cycles. Hundreds of eggs vanish each month, and by the time of the menopause only about 1000 are left.

The change of life should occur gradually, allowing the body to adapt to its new condition with ease. Because a woman ceases to ovulate, she no longer produces progesterone, so the body compensates by sending a message to the pituitary gland to release increased quantities of FSH and LH.

The onset of the menopause is commonly confirmed by a rise in the levels of these two hormones in the blood (see Fig. 4 below).

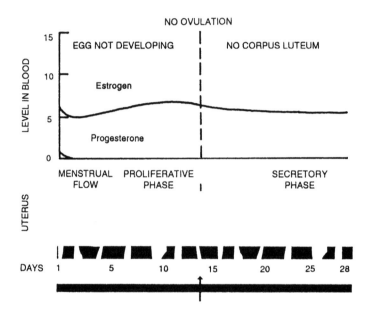

Figure 4 – The menopause

PART 2

HORMONES IN HAVOC

CHAPTER 2

....

THE RISE OF HORMONAL HEALTH PROBLEMS

Something is seriously amiss with our hormones. Over the last 50 years there's been an undeniable escalation in hormone-related health problems. The incidence of infertility, fibroids, endometriosis, polycystic breasts, ovarian, cervical and breast cancer have increased steadily and dramatically. As nutrition consultants, we cannot help but notice the rise in these problems. Even more worryingly, many hormone-related diseases are occurring earlier in life. Complaints like endometriosis, fibroids and ovarian cysts used to be extremely rare in teenage girls but they are now quite common and sometimes result in irreversible infertility.

The reality of the hormonal havoc we now face, especially in the Western world, becomes vividly clear when we look at cancer statistics. Cancer is a condition in which certain body cells start to misbehave, growing and multiplying rapidly with complete disregard for the territory of neighboring cells. Cancer occurs in a variety of locations and types of tissues. Some of these tissues are known to be very hormone-sensitive. An example is breast tissue. While some non-hormone related cancers are not increasing greatly (lung cancer, for example, is on the decline), hormone-related cancers are very much on the rise. The probability of a person developing these hormone-related cancers during their life is shown below, comparing actual figures in 1985 with predicted figures in the years 2000, and 2015.[1]

Cancer Incidence and Risk

	1985	2000	2015
Breast (women)	8.6%	9.1%	11.6%
Uterine (women)	1.2%	1.8%	2.2%
Prostate (men)	7.1%	13.5%	23.7%
Testicular (men)	0.4%	0.4%	0.6%

The incidence of breast cancer, for example, has nearly tripled in the last 30 years.

The problems don't just relate to women. Rates of testicular and prostate cancer are shooting up, with prostate cancer predicted to more than double in the next 20 years.

THE EARLY SIGNS OF HORMONAL HAVOC

While hormonal cancers may be seen as the end result of substantial and probably long-term changes in hormonal health, the early warning signs are undeniable. The number of boys born with genital defects or undescended testes has doubled. More girls are now reaching maturity at nine. According to Dr Marcia Herman-Giddens of the University of North Carolina, whose research found that 48 per cent of black girls and 15 per cent of white girls were developing breasts and pubic hair before their tenth birthdays: 'All of us in pediatric practice had a sense that girls were developing earlier, but we were still surprised at how young many of them were.'[2] Puberty onset has dropped to an average of 11 years old, compared with an average of 17 in Victorian girls and 13 in the 1970s. These changes are particularly concerning since early onset of puberty is associated with an increased risk of breast cancer and menopausal problems.

PMS – IS IT IN THE MIND?

Women's suffering hasn't always been taken that seriously in medical history, and there is no better example of this than premenstrual syndrome (PMS), the symptoms of which include breast tenderness, fatigue, bloating, headaches, mood swings, depression, irritability and fatigue. These are symptoms of a hormonal imbalance now thought to affect 74 per cent of women. Two surveys by the Women's Nutritional Advisory Service – one in 1985, the other in 1996 – show that the severity of PMS is increasing.[3] In the 1996 survey, mood swings, depression, anxiety and aggressive feelings were experienced by 80 per cent of sufferers premenstrually, and 52 per cent had contemplated suicide in their premenstrual phase.

Yet some psychologists still argue that PMS doesn't exist, saying it's all in the mind. According to Dr Marion Stewart from the Women's Nutritional Advisory Service, PMS (at least on the scale that it is now experienced) is a twentieth-century disease – the result of poor nutrition and increased levels of stress due to the changing role of women in modern society. These symptoms completely disappear in 90 per cent of women within four months of changing their diet, doing some exercise and finding effective ways of dealing with stress.

ENDOMETRIOSIS – THE HIDDEN EPIDEMIC

Endometriosis – a condition in which cells like those lining the uterus begin to grow on other organs of the body where they do not belong – is being diagnosed in more and more women in their early teens and twenties. One in 10 women in their reproductive years, from 11 to 60, is affected.[4] Symptoms vary but may include severe period pain, heavy bleeding, pain on menstruation or pain with intercourse. The pain can be so severe as to be totally debilitating, affecting a woman's ability to lead a normal, fulfilling life. Loss of fertility is investigated in at least half of those with endometriosis as 30 to 40 per cent of sufferers cannot conceive; it is a major cause of infertility and is present in up to 43 per cent of infertile women. Although endometriosis is not a new condition, evidence suggests that it too is on the increase.

BEWARE THOSE LUMPS

Much more common than breast cancer is breast lumps, known as polycystic or fibrocystic breast disease. These occur in at least 25 per cent of women at some time in their lives. More often than not, these lumps are not malignant (cancer-producing). However the risk of developing breast cancer is higher in those with a history of breast lumps.

Even more common are fibroids (growths in the uterus). They often grow to the size of a grapefruit and can cause irregular, heavy and painful periods. The incidence of fibroids and cysts on the ovaries, thought to result from disrupted ovulation, have both increased, probably as a consequence of hormonal imbalance.

A GOOD SPERM IS HARD TO FIND

In case you're thinking women have a raw deal, men have hormonal problems too. While they may not have to worry about PMS or lumps, men do have a menopause with very similar symptoms to women. According to male hormone expert Dr Malcolm Carruthers, the symptoms of the male menopause (known as the andropause) include fatigue, depression, irritability, rapid aging, aches and pains, sweating and flashing, and decreased sexual performance. Having treated thousands of men, Dr Carruthers, author of *The Male Menopause*, is convinced that the andropause is real and rapidly on the increase.[5] Those most at risk, according to his research, are farmers, due to their frequent exposure to organophosphate in sheep dip, pesticides and other agro-chemicals, including hormones used in intensive animal rearing.

However, according to Dr Niels Shakkebaek, a repro-ductive scientist for the World Health Organization, many symptom-free men are also showing signs of hormonal and sexual imbalance. After analysing the data from over 60 scientific studies in the last 50 years, involving almost 15,000 men, he concluded that the average sperm count had dropped by 50 per cent in five decades.[6] However, it wasn't just the quantity but also the quality that had fallen, with a lower percentage of healthy sperm able to fertilize an egg.

Men are also facing a rapid escalation in the risk of testicu-lar and prostate cancer, as well as prostate disease. The prostate is a ring-shaped gland, about the size of a chestnut, that lies under the bladder and surrounds the top of the ure-thra (urine duct) in men. Its job is to secrete a slightly acidic fluid that contributes to seminal fluid and improves the motil-ity and viability of sperm. If it is enlarged (a condition known as benign prostatic hyperplasia – BPH), or affected by benign or malignant tumors, it can act like a clamp and impede the flow of urine. BPH is unlikely to be a topic of conversation at your next dinner party – indeed one in ten men with BPH actively avoids consulting his doctor about the problem. It develops after the age of 40 and affects about one-third of all men over the age of 60 – that's about two million men in the UK, resulting in 40,000 prostate operations in the UK every year.

While there appears to be no direct correlation, both BPH

and prostate cancer are very much on the increase. Prostate cancer is the fastest-growing cancer and is predicted to affect one in four men within 20 years.

ONE IN SEVEN COUPLES IS INFERTILE

While the average sperm count fell from 113 million per ml in 1940 to 66 million in 1990, levels below 20 million per ml are associated with infertility. Dr Skakkebaek and others have found that an increasing number of men have these low levels of viable sperm. Professor Louis Guillette, a respected reproductive expert, concluded, 'Today's man is half the man his grandfather was." While men account for an estimated 40 per cent of cases of infertility, it is likely that increasing hormonal problems in both men and women are responsible for the gradual decline in overall fertility; so much so, that about one in seven couples is currently infertile. If the fall in sperm count continues, one might expect rates of infertility to escalate rapidly when sperm counts reach half their current average, posing a hitherto unthought of threat to the human race.

When we put all the pieces of the puzzle together it is hard to deny that, as we approach the twenty-first century, we are having trouble keeping our hormones balanced. The question is why? Are these problems connected or not? And what are the solutions? The next chapter follows some leads in one of the most extraordinary detective stories of our time.

CHAPTER 3

....

THE FEMINIZATION OF
NATURE

One big clue to the underlying causes of hormone imbalance was first brought to the public's attention by Theo Colborn, a scientist working for the World Wildlife Research Fund in Washington.[7] She had been recording bizarre changes in health and behavior in a wide variety of different species. Disrupted mating, rearing behavior and fertility were being reported all around the world. Alligators in Lake Apopka in Florida had all but stopped producing eggs during the 1980s, threatening their survival. On investigation, 60 per cent of the males had shrunken genitals. Herring gulls in Lake Ontario were abandoning their nests, leaving unhatched eggs and deformed chicks. Female gulls were setting up nests with other female gulls. In 1988, off the coasts of Sweden, Denmark, Scotland and Ireland, the seal population seemed to be dying off. Aborted seals were being washed ashore. In 1990 a similar problem affected dolphins in the Mediterranean. These last two examples had the hallmarks of an infectious epidemic, but what was making these animals so susceptible? Why were so many species, including man, showing tell-tale signs of hormone disruption and failing fertility?

DDT AND PCBs – A DANGEROUS LEGACY

As these natural anomalies were investigated, a pattern started to emerge. All the affected species contained high levels of chemical contaminants, such as DDT, DDE or PCBs (polychlorinated biphenyls). These chemicals don't biodegrade and, although DDT has been banned in most countries for at least 20 years, its concentration seems to have been accumulating along the food chain. Both Lake Apopka and Lake Ontario had become contaminated. In Lake Ontario, plankton was found to contain 250 parts of PCBs; smelt, which fed off this, had 835,000; lake trout had 2,800,000 parts; while the herring gull, which fed off the lake trout, had 25,000,000 parts. Like seals and humans, the herring gull was at the end of a polluted food chain.

While organochlorine pesticides, such as DDT, are rarely used any more in the UK, an analysis of human fat (an indicator of our ability to accumulate less biodegradable pesticides), performed in 1995, found DDT in 99 per cent of fat samples, with a quarter of samples containing amounts between 1 and 9mg per kg.[8]

Conventional scientific wisdom would say that these levels are very low and don't represent a health hazard, yet three pieces of research have radically changed the way we understand the power of these and other hormone-disrupting chemicals. The first was the work of Frederick vom Saal, a professor of biology at the University of Missouri.[9] He knew a lot about mice and had observed that about one in six female mice behaved in a much more aggressive and "masculinized" way. He wondered why. His research proved that, during fetal development, if a female pup lay between two males in the uterus, she developed these "male" characteristics. It seemed the tiny changes in exposure to the male hormones of the pup's neighbors had the power to program the female mouse for her entire life.

Meanwhile, a number of independent researchers have demonstrated that exposing animals during fetal development to tiny amounts of DDT or PCBs has significant effects on their development, often stimulating genital defects, infertility, low sperm counts, early puberty, higher rates of certain cancers, weakened immune systems and disrupted sexual behavior – a remarkably similar set of symptoms to those being recorded in humans.

OTHER HORMONE-DISRUPTING CHEMICALS

As research continues, an increasingly wide variety of chemicals is being found to have hormone-disrupting properties. Many of these are present in tiny amounts in all of us; you'd probably find that your blood contained at least 250 identifiable contaminants if you spent the money on tests. But the levels are generally so low as to be of little concern on their own. However, more and more studies are indicating that the combination of tiny amounts of hormone-disrupting chemicals has an even more sinister effect that the sum of the effects of the individual chemicals.

Maybe the rapid increase in hormone- and immune-related health problems is the result of small, yet significant changes in our exposure to these hormone-disrupting chemicals, especially in the uterus and early life. According to Deborah Cadbury, author of *The Feminization of Nature*, leading scientists from many disciplines have come to the same conclusions.

"We've released chemicals throughout the world that are having fundamental effects on the reproductive system and immune system in wildlife and humans," says Professor Louis Guillette from the University of Florida.

"We have unwittingly entered the ultimate Faustian bargain . . . In return for all the benefits of our modern society, and all the amazing products of modern life, we have more testicular cancer and more breast cancer. We may also affect the ability of the species to reproduce," says Devra Lee Davis, former deputy health policy advisor to the American government.

They, and countless other scientists, have come to the conclusion that a growing number of commonly occurring chemicals found in air, water and food are disrupting our hormonal balance and altering the course of nature. What these chemicals are, and what you can do to avoid them, is the subject of the next chapter.

CHAPTER 4

THE SEA OF ESTROGENS

Our modern chemical world is very different from that of our ancestors. There are now 100,000 synthetic chemicals on the international market, including 15,000 chlorinated compounds such as PCBs. Some of these are put directly into food; others are added indirectly, in the form of pesticide residues or accumulation up the food chain from non-biodegradable industrial contaminants. Some creep into our food from packaging and processing. Some we take as medicine.

These hormone-disrupting chemicals include:

- **Pesticides** – DDT, DDE, endosulfan, methoxychlor, heptachlor, toxaphene, dieldrin, lindane

- **Plastic compounds** – alkyphenols, such as nonylphenol and octylphenol; biphenolic compounds, such as bisphenol A; phthalates

- **Industrial compounds** – some PCBs, dioxin; plus those listed for plastics

- **Pharmaceutical drugs** – synthetic estrogens, such as DES

Most of these mimic the role of estrogen in our bodies, stimulating the growth of hormone-sensitive tissue. When combined with the natural estrogen produced by both men and women, plus the added estrogen taken in by women on the Pill or HRT, these chemicals can "over-estrogenize" a person. Too much estrogen stimulates the excessive proliferation of hormone-sensitive tissue, thus increasing the risk of hormone-related cancers. The effect of these chemicals is not, however, quite so direct. Essentially they confuse the hormonal messages the body sends out, changing our sexual and reproductive development. They are best thought of as hormone-disrupters, interfering with the body's ability to adapt and respond to its environment.

Such worldwide increased exposure to these hormone-disrupters is even more worrying in the light of the finding that a very small change in hormone exposure during fetal development can lead to infertility and increased cancer risk in adulthood. In other words, these chemicals are programming us for extinction.

Another troubling development is that girls seem to be reaching puberty earlier. The first signs of sexual maturity are now frequently appearing in younger children and, according to Professor Richard Sharpe of the Medical Research Council, "If you expose animals to low levels of extra estrogen neonatally, they will have advanced puberty."

ANTI-ADAPTOGENS

These chemicals, and the broad spectrum of ill-effects they appear to be generating, can be seen as anti-adaptogens, interfering with our innate ability to adapt to our environment. They are a spanner in the works of our endocrine and immune systems whose job is to ensure that we adapt our body systems to maintain good health. Coupled with a poor intake of adaptogens – vitamins, minerals, essential fats and phytonutrients – which help to balance our hormones and increase our ability to adapt, these chemicals are leading us towards disaster in terms of ever-decreasing hormonal health.

Such substances are thought to disrupt the body's bio-chemistry because of their ability to lock on to hormone receptor sites. This alters the ability of genes to communicate with the body's cells (gene expression), which is vital for the orchestration of health. In some cases these chemicals block a hormone receptor; in other cases they act as if they were the hormone; and some simply disrupt the hormone message. If you think of this "hormone→ hormone receptor→ gene expression→ biochemical response" sequence as "communication," what such chemicals do is turn the "sound" up or down and scramble the message. This is because they do not fit the receptor site perfectly. Our body's chemistry hasn't been exposed to them before and hasn't managed to adapt its response accordingly.

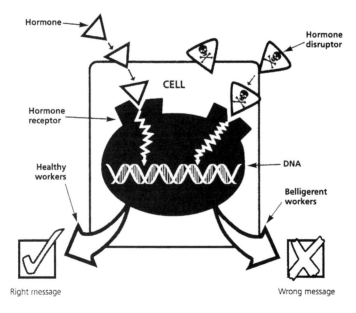

Figure 5 – How hormones and chemicals affect genes

THE TROUBLE WITH SYNTHETIC HORMONES

The same is true of synthetic hormones. Take progesterone, for example, which is a hormone that is naturally produced by the body. It has a precise chemical structure: only this exact molecule can trigger a particular set of instructions which maintain pregnancy, bone density, normal menstruation and other steps in the hormonal dance that occurs in every woman. It has, even at levels considerably higher than those produced by the human body, remarkably little toxicity.

Yet, almost without exception, every contraceptive pill or HRT prescription – pill, patch or depot (a deposition of hormones under the skin which release over time) – contains synthetic progestins, altered molecules that are similar to, but different from, genuine progesterone. They are like keys that open the lock, but don't fit exactly; consequently they generate a wobble in the biochemistry of the body. Not surprisingly, toxicity increases – so much so that the side-effects include increased risk of diseases such as breast cancer, against which the natural molecule actually protects us.

The same applies to estrogen, or more correctly, estrogens. Unlike progesterone, there is a family of naturally produced estrogens – the main three are estriol, estrone and estradiol. During pregnancy, estriol is produced in significantly larger quantities than at other times, when estrone and estradiol pre-dominate. Many pharmaceutical drugs, including contraceptive pills and HRT, use synthetic estrogens which mimic the effects of these naturally occurring molecules.

There could be no more dramatic example of the danger of altering our exposure to these powerful hormone-mimickers than DES, the first synthetic estrogen, created by Dr Charles Dodds in 1938. Within 20 years, DES was being given to women and to animals. For the latter it improved growth rates, while for women it apparently promised a trouble-free pregnancy and healthier offspring. Eventually, up to six million mothers and babies were exposed to DES. It wasn't until 1970 that the problems surfaced. Girls whose mothers had been on DES during pregnancy started to show abnormal genital development and a substantial increase in cancer rates, especially vaginal cancer of a kind never seen before. It was then discovered that boys of mothers who had taken DES also had defects in the development of sexual organs. Many DES children even died and many more were infertile.

The danger of synthetic hormones doesn't just lie in the subtle differences in their chemical structure and effect, but also in the amounts given and their relative balance with other hormones. The level of hormones in a contraceptive pill or HRT treatment may be many times higher than the body would naturally produce. Estrogen produced by the body is balanced with progesterone but, if this balance is lost (and estrogen is no longer opposed by progesterone), health problems arise. It is unopposed estrogen, rather than estrogen per se, that seems to be the problem.

UNOPPOSED ESTROGEN LINKED TO CANCER

Excessive exposure to estrogen and estrogen-mimickers may be a major factor in hormone-related cancers. If breast epithelial cells are exposed to estrogen, their rate of abnormal proliferation doubles. A study by Dr Bergkvist and colleagues in Scandinavia showed that if a woman is on HRT for longer than five years she doubles her risk of breast cancer.[10] They also found that if the HRT included progestins (the synthetic versions of natural progesterone) that risk was even higher.

A large-scale study, published in the *New England Journal of Medicine* in 1995, showed that post-menopausal women who had been on HRT for five or more years had a 71 per cent increased risk of breast cancer.[11] The risk was found to increase with length of time on HRT. Overall, there was a 32 per cent increased risk among women using estrogen HRT, and a 41 per cent risk for those using estrogen and synthetic progestin HRT, compared to women who had never used hormones. Another study in 1995 carried out by the Emery University School for Public Health, followed 240,000 women for eight years; results showed that the risk of ovarian cancer was 72 per cent higher in women given estrogen.[12] According to Dr John Lee, medical expert in female hormones and health, from California, "The major cause of breast cancer is unopposed estrogen and there are many factors that would lead to this. Xenoestrogens [synthetic, estrogen-like compounds, found in plastics etc] have the ability to damage tissue and lead to an increased risk of cancer later in life. There are also clearly nutritional and genetic factors to consider. What is most concerning is that doctors continue to prescribe unopposed estrogen to women."[13]

DIETARY ESTROGENS

We also take in estrogens from natural food. Meat contains significant amounts of estrogen, as does dairy produce. However, the high levels in these foods may indicate that they aren't perhaps as natural as we like to think. Much of the meat we eat comes from animals whose feed contains added hormones. This, coupled with a high protein intake, forces the growth of the animal, which means more profit. Changes in farming practices now make it possible to milk cows continuously, even while they are pregnant. Milk taken from a pregnant cow contains substantially more estrogen.

Meat and dairy products also store up non-degradable toxins which accumulate along the food chain. Millions of tons of chemicals, like non-biodegradable PCBs and DDT, have been released into the environment. Traces of these non-degradable chemicals are found in meat, fish and fowl, which have fed on other animals who have fed on contaminated pastures or water; the chemicals accumulate in fat and, when we eat animal fat, they accumulate in us.

Plants also contain estrogen-like compounds, known as phyto-estrogens. These are found in a wide variety of foods including soya, citrus fruits, wheat, licorice, alfalfa, celery and fennel. The richest source is soya and soya products such as tofu or soya milk. However, unlike estrogenic chemicals such as PCBs, these phyto-estrogens are associated with a reduced risk of cancer. A high dietary intake of isoflavones, the active ingredient in soya, is associated with a halving of breast cancer in animals, and a substantial reduction in deaths from prostate cancer in men. There is no clear explanation of this anomaly, although two theories exist. One is that these naturally occurring phyto-estrogens may act as adaptogens. That is, they help the body stabilize hormone levels. The other is that they may block the action of other more toxic environmental estrogens, perhaps by occupying the receptor sites. Even more encouraging are animal studies which show that eating a small amount of isoflavones in early infancy results in a 60 per cent reduced risk of breast cancer later in life.

While the effects of consuming phyto-estrogens seem to be all positive, there is some cause for concern over taking in very large amounts during the critical early years of development, which is exactly what would occur if an infant were bottle-fed using a soya-based formula. No one really knows if this is potentially beneficial or detrimental for hormonal health later in life because no research has yet been done. What can be said is that it is no more natural for an infant to be fed soya milk than it is to be fed cow's milk. There is no substitute to good quality human breast milk for infants.

CHAPTER 5

THE STRESS CONNECTION

Another way to upset your hormone balance is by eating the wrong kind of food and being permanently stressed. We produce many different hormones that keep the body in balance. These include insulin and glucagon to keep our blood sugar level even; adrenalin and cortisol to help us react to stress; thyroxine which controls our rate of metabolism; the sex hormones discussed in Part 1; and a whole host of hormones produced by the pituitary gland in the center of the head that effectively conducts the hormonal orchestra of our bodies.

Whenever you take in a stimulant such as coffee or a cigarette, or react stressfully to an event, the body produces the adrenal hormone cortisol. This competes for receptor sites with progesterone. So the net effect of being permanently in a stressed or stimulated state is less active progesterone. Since cortisol also increases the production of estrogen, prolonged stress can contribute to estrogen dominance. Normally the liver can easily deal with slight excesses of estrogen; if, however, a person's diet is poor, or they have allergies, or take in excessive toxins, the liver's ability to detoxify and eliminate estrogen can be impaired.

Stress also upsets the balance of the "male hormone," as some testosterone is made by the adrenal glands in women as well as men. A disturbance in the balance of male and female hormones in women can lead to a lack of ovulation and the development of excessive facial hair and other male characteristics.

STRESS AND BLOOD SUGAR CONTROL

The net result of stress, or a diet too high in sugar and refined carbohydrates, is an inability to keep blood sugar levels stable, known as dysglycemia. When blood sugar levels shoot up, after sugar intake, a stimulant or a stressful reaction, the body has to produce more insulin to get the sugar out of the blood and into the body cells. When the blood sugar level is too low this stimulates the adrenal hormone cortisol. This sort of disturbed hormone balance has many undesirable knock-on effects on health, including a greater risk of PMS, polycystic ovaries, and an under-active thyroid gland (leading to weight gain, fatigue and sluggishness). Ninety per cent of those with polycystic ovarian syndrome show this kind of hormone imbalance. No doubt it also contributes to many other female health problems.

This pattern of dysglycemia, with raised insulin and cortisol levels is known as "syndrome X" and increases the risk of inflammatory health problems. While one might think of arthritis, asthma and eczema as involving inflammation, so too do atherosclerosis (disease of the arteries), diabetes and Alzheimer's. This may explain why post-menopausal women (who still produce some estrogen but no progesterone) have a much greater risk of cardiovascular disease than pre-menopausal women.

STRESS AND WEIGHT GAIN

Syndrome X may also be the reason why some women experience weight gain despite no apparent increase in calories consumed. Dr Kate Steinbeck and colleagues at the Royal

Prince Albert Hospital in Sydney found that children who have "syndrome X" have, in later life, a greater propensity to turn food into fat, as well as a greater risk of diabetes and heart disease.

Hormone imbalances brought on by the wrong kind of diet, lifestyle and exposure to hormone-disrupting chemicals, can also lead to either an androgen (masculinizing hormones) dominance or estrogen dominance. Excessive androgen levels are now being linked to upper body and waist weight gain, while high estrogen (feminizing hormone) levels are associated with lower body weight gain. For this reason, "apple-shaped" people may be more likely to be androgen dominant, a factor associated with blood sugar problems and syndrome X, while "pear-shaped" people may be more likely to be estrogen dominant. Either way, too much stress, sugar and stimulants are likely to make matters worse.

CHAPTER 6

....

THE WAY BACK TO HEALTH

You have probably realized by now that your diet, environment and lifestyle are all factors that can rock the boat of your hormonal health. If the load gets too great, the boat tips over and hormone-related diseases may ensue. Once this happens, ignorance is *not* bliss. Armed with a good understanding of how to tip the odds in your favor, there is a lot you can do to protect, maintain and improve your health. The first step is to avoid the hormone-disrupters.

AVOIDING THE HORMONE-DISRUPTERS

Why, you may ask, don't we just ban all these hormone-disrupting chemicals? As Professor Louis Guillette, from the University of Florida, says, "Should we change policy? Should we be upset? I think we should be fundamentally upset. I think we should be screaming in the streets." Yet, the reality, until large-scale government action is taken, is that it isn't easy to eliminate all these substances because they are all around us – in our food, water, air and household products. There are, however, steps you can take to substantially reduce your own and your family's exposure.

First of all, you can buy organic produce wherever possible and avoid using pesticides or herbicides in your own garden or home. This immediately cuts down your exposure. It's not a bad idea to cut back on meat and dairy produce, or, at least, choose organic meat when you do eat it.

Plastic is impossible and unnecessary to avoid. It is, however, worth reducing your exposure to food in contact with plastic, particularly if the food is hot, liquid or acidic. This is because some soft plastics use plasticizers such as nonylphenol or bisphenol A which do disrupt hormones and can pass into the foods. Examples of this may include packaged TV dinners destined for the microwave; and some tins of food or juice cartons which are lined with plastic. Check the foods you buy. Choose juice in glass bottles or unlined cans whenever possible. Use cling-film sparingly, if at all. Put your sandwiches in a brown bag rather than cling-film. Also, check household and cosmetic products you buy for the following chemicals: bisphenol-A, octoxynol, nonoxynol, noylphenol, octylphenol and ethoxylate.

Think carefully before going on the Pill or taking HRT. These are discussed fully in Part 4. Avoid excess sugar, stimulants and stress, as explained in the last chapter.

Some general guidelines are summarized below:

- **Eat organic.** This instantly minimizes your exposure to pesticides and herbicides. When you are eating non-organic produce wash it in an acidic medium, made by adding 1 tablespoon vinegar to a bowl of water. This will reduce some, but not all, pesticides.

- **Filter all drinking water.** We recommend getting a water filter installed under the sink, made from stainless steel, not plastic or aluminium, and employing some kind of carbon-filtration system. While not proven to remove all hormone-disrupting chemicals, this should decrease your load. The alternative is spring water, bottled in glass.

- **Reduce your intake of fatty foods.** Non-biodegradable chemicals accumulate up the food chain in animal fat.

Minimizing your intake of animal fat, (meat and dairy produce) lessens your exposure. There is no need to limit essential fats in nuts and seeds.

- **Never heat food in plastic.*** This means saying goodbye to microwaved TV dinners. If you have to have them, transfer the food into a glass container before heating.

- **Minimize fatty foods in plastic.*** Some chemicals that keep plastics flexible easily pass out of the plastic into fatty foods; including crisps, cheese, butter, chocolate and pies.

- **Minimize liquid foods in plastic.*** This not only includes fruit juices in cardboard packs, which have a plastic inner lining, but also some canned fruits and vegetables, which may also have a plastic inner lining.

- **Minimize exposure of food to plastic.*** This means using paper bags to put your vegetables in, as opposed to buying everything in plastic trays, covered with cling-film.

- **Switch to natural detergents.** Use only ecological detergent products, for washing up, washing clothes and body washing from companies who declare all their ingredients. Also, rinse well after washing up.

- **Don't use pesticides in your garden.** Some pesticides are hormone-disrupters. Unless you're sure yours isn't, it is better not to spray. Research is suggesting a link between higher rates of childhood cancer and homes whose gardens are sprayed with pesticides.

- **Don't use the contraceptive pill or HRT.** There are many safer ways to avoid conception and restore hormonal health (explained in detail in Part 4).

---

* Until the plastics industry either stops using all suspect chemicals, or discloses which chemicals are contained in their products, you have no way of knowing if hormone-disrupting chemicals are present or not.

PART 3

BALANCING HORMONES NATURALLY

CHAPTER 7

....

OPTIMUM NUTRITION – THE KEY TO HORMONE BALANCE

Hormones are made from the foods you eat. Eating the right food is therefore essential for forming and balancing your hormones. If you supply your body with second-rate fuel then it will, over time, give you second-rate performance. But it isn't just what you eat that determines your health, it's also how well you digest it.

The digestive tract is in fact the largest endocrine gland in the body, producing many hormones that work with the nervous system to control digestion and absorption. The digestive tract (which, if laid flat, would occupy an area the size of a small football pitch) takes each morsel of ingested food through three processes: the breakdown of food into simple units – digestion; the transport of nutrients across the gut wall into the blood – absorption; and the selective ejection of waste – elimination.

Giving the digestive tract low-grade fuel puts undue strain on the system; your body is geared for survival, not destruction. The extra effort required to deal with inappropriate foods is wasted energy and draws on your body's reserves of nutrients in an attempt to cope – valuable nutrients that would be better spent balancing your energy, mood and hormones.

According to nutrition expert Dr Abram Hoffer, "Modern diets are designed to appeal to the senses. Modern food bears little relationship to our physiological needs. Modern high tech food processing has robbed us of the use of our senses in determining whether a food is or is not good for us."

It is only recently that it has become necessary to educate ourselves about the composition of food. Our ancestors learnt very effectively which foods were safe to eat by trial and error. Foods that were bland, salty or sweet were preferred, and, as a rule, are not poisonous. These were balanced wholefoods needed to maintain health. Today our food supplies have been manipulated in such a way that we no longer recognize what is and what is not a healthy food.

For example, many of us now consider that good-quality fruit and vegetables will be uniform in shape and size and bear no blemishes. We go into supermarkets and see rows and rows of apples all looking the same (the average apple having been sprayed with chemicals around 25 times). Nowhere in nature do you find such uniformity, but we have grown accustomed to it and see the rather misshapen, organically grown alternative as unsavory.

Detoxifying hormones

The body has to expend energy detoxifying every man-made chemical, pollutant or inappropriate food that goes into it. Yet every process in the body, especially detoxification, depends on nutrients such as vitamins and minerals. The problem with man-made chemicals, pollutants and inappropriate foods is that they either do not supply any nutrients or may require even more to detoxify them than they provide in the first place. This leads to ever-increasing nutritional depletion and impaired detoxification potential.

Hormones have to be detoxified, as do the hormone-like substances we inadvertently take in from pesticides, plastics and detergent residues. If they are not, imbalances such as estrogen dominance, are created. Eating the wrong foods and living in a state of stress can play havoc with the digestive system. Sometimes, even after a long period on a good diet, the long-term damaging effects of stress and poor diet on the digestive tract are not entirely reversed. As nutrition consultants, we treat the digestive tract with a great deal of respect, knowing that if it is not functioning well there is little chance that the rest of the body will be able to perform well.

THE PROBLEMS OF DIGESTION

In order to deal with food, good or bad, the digestive processes need to be in good working order. The first major obstacle is when the food reaches the stomach. Here the body starts to digest the complex proteins mainly found in animal produce, nuts, seeds, pulses and grains. Conditions in the stomach need to be very acid in order to break down the complex proteins. Zinc is required to make the conditions in the stomach sufficiently acid. In fact, the body has a high demand for zinc, which is involved in over 200 reactions: it is required at every step of the reproductive process and is used in vast amounts when we are stressed. When the acid in the stomach starts to work on the proteins, the minerals are freed up, ready for absorption. A lack of acid can impair mineral absorption.

The symptoms of low acid are similar to having too much acid, mainly indigestion and heartburn. Many women over 50 do not produce enough stomach acid and are commonly prescribed antacids which further deplete production. Rarely are they given any dietary advice: taking antacids and continuing to eat a high protein diet is only likely to compound the problem.

Poor digestion leads to larger than expected particles of food entering the bowels. The larger particles of food can act as local irritants on the gut wall, contributing to increased permeability, commonly called "leaky gut syndrome." When larger particles of food enter the large bowel, the home of the microflora, the bacteria residing there feed off the unexpected feast and create flatulence and bloating.

LEAKY GUT SYNDROME

If the gut wall becomes leakier than it should, three main problems may arise. A healthy gut has a specific permeability that allows for the transfer of nutrients – digested proteins, fats and carbohydrates, and vitamins, minerals, phyto-nutrients and water. Man-made chemicals, like pesticides, may also get across a normal gut wall, as can heavy metals like lead and cadmium, particularly if our intake of essential minerals like calcium, magnesium and zinc is low or our consumption of alcohol is high.

Problem 1 – Increased risk of food allergy: If larger particles of food enter the small intestine and irritate the gut wall, making it leakier, then they are able to cross over into the bloodstream. The immune system sees larger particles of food as foreign and triggers an allergic reaction (see Chapter 16). Prolonged stress also suppresses proper immune system function in the digestive tract.

Problem 2 – Decreased mineral absorption: Contrary to what one may have thought, if the gut becomes more permeable its ability to absorb minerals is reduced. This is because minerals are normally picked up actively by a protein carrier and taken across the gut wall into the blood. When the gut wall is damaged the carrier proteins are also damaged. This, combined with a low level of stomach acid, and high exposure to pollutants and alcohol, is especially bad news for nutrient absorption. Alcohol can also destroy B vitamins in the gut. On top of this, if your diet is high in wheat and soya, two major sources of phytates in food, then the problem is further compounded, as phytates are capable of binding with minerals such as calcium, iron and zinc, preventing them from being properly absorbed. Caffeine from coffee and tannin from tea rob the body of the same minerals.

Problem 3 – Increased risk of absorbing toxins: If the gut is of normal permeability then most toxins don't get through. Nature did not design the digestive tract to be permeable to toxins, but when the gut becomes leakier than it should they can be absorbed into the blood more readily.

The common causes, besides incompletely digested food particles, of the gut becoming too "leaky" are:

- prolonged stress
- excessive growth of candidiasis
- certain drugs, including synthetic hormones, chemo-therapeutic agents, and non-steroidal anti-inflammatory drugs which irritate the digestive tract
- surgery and radiotherapy
- infection, especially gut infections
- regular ingestion of alcohol
- nutritional deficiencies leading to a weakened gut wall
- inflammatory bowel disorders such as IBS or colitis
- impaired immune function

A simple urine test can identify whether your gut is of normal permeability or not. Nutrition consultants can recommend this test for you. In our practice we have picked up problems with absorption time and time again, even among people who are eating reasonably well. Some clients of ours who had been following nutritional programs for a year or more had certainly got a lot better but were not always as well as they hoped. After measuring acid production, digestive enzyme production and gut permeability, we commonly found either a problem with digestion, gut permeability or both. When we treated these directly with specific agents, their health took another quantum leap. We also found low vitamin and mineral status, despite the fact that they were following a good nutritional program. After four to six months on a digestive program, not only were these levels within a normal range, but their digestive profiles were also normal. We have continued to have this success with hundreds of clients since.

So, if you suffer from heartburn, indigestion, flatulence, bloating, diarrhea or constipation or any other digestive problems, it is well worth checking how well your digestive processes are working, particularly if you believe that you have been eating well and supplementing nutrients for some time.

HEALTHY DIGESTION – THE KEY TO HORMONAL HEALTH

We cannot emphasize enough how important the digestive tract is in achieving hormonal balance and optimum health. Many of the symptoms attributed to sex hormone imbalances, such as irritability, anxiety, depression, lack of energy, joint pains, water retention, weight gain and bloating, have their origins in digestive problems.

Blood sugar imbalance, food allergies, candidiasis (the yeast organism responsible for causing thrush) and stress can all give rise to symptoms often associated with hormonal imbalances. Unless you already know that you have a sex hormone imbalance, we recommend that you pay special attention to Chapters 15, 16 and 17 before you assume that an imbalance in your sex hormones is the cause of your symptoms. In so many cases, when women address these issues, their health problems clear up. Even those women with true sex hormone imbalances do very much better when they take these factors into account.

We only recommend the use of natural hormones when there is already a diagnosed sex hormone imbalance that would warrant this, after all dietary strategies have been fully explored and hormone imbalances have been tested, as described in Part 4.

The following Hormonal Health Questionnaire can help you identify which underlying factors may be affecting your health.

Hormonal Health Questionnaire

For any question to which your answer is "yes" highlight the entire box in the column to the right.

- Do you use the contraceptive pill? — | | | C | H |
- In the last five years have you taken antibiotics for one month, or longer or shorter courses four or more times a year? — | | | C | |
- Do you ever experience joint pains? — | A | | C | H |
- Do you experience water retention? — | A | | | |
- Is it cyclical? — | | | | H |
- Are your symptoms worse on damp or muggy days or in mouldy places? — | | | C | |
- Do you ever suffer from headaches? — | A | | C | |
- Do they happen after eating? — | | G | | |
- Are they often cyclical? — | | | | H |
- Do you have excess hair on your body or thinning hair on your scalp? — | | | | H |
- Have you gained weight on your upper body? — | | G | | |
- Have you gained weight on your thighs and hips? — | | | | H |
- Do you often suffer from mood swings? — | A | G | C | H |

- Are they often cyclical?

			H

- Do you suffer from fatigue or drowsiness during the day?

A	G	C	H

- Are you slow to wake up in the morning?

A	G		

- Do you suffer from insomnia?

A	G	C	H

- Do you easily become irritable?

A	G	C	H

- Do you suffer from memory loss or poor concentration?

A	G	C	H

- Do you suffer from depression?

A		C	H

- Is it often cyclical?

			H

- Do you suffer from flatulence or bloating?

A		C	H

- Do you suffer from food cravings?

A	G	C	

- Do you especially crave foods premenstrually?

			H

- Are you addicted to sweet foods?

	G	C	

- Do you experience excessive thirst?

A	G		

- Do you become irritable without food?

A	G	C	

- Have you at any time been bothered with problems affecting your reproductive organs?

		C	H

- Do you have trouble conceiving or a history of miscarriage?

			H

- Do you suffer from breast tenderness?

			H

- Do you experience cramps or other menstrual irregularities?

		C	H

- Are your periods often irregular or heavy?

			H

- Do you suffer from lumpy breasts?

			H

- Do you suffer from reduced libido?

A	G	C	H

- Do you often suffer from thrush?

		C	H

- Do you have any known allergies?

A			

- Does exposure to perfumes, odors or chemicals
  affect you?

		C	

- Do you suffer from irritable bowel syndrome?

A		C	

- Do you suffer from constipation?

A			H

- Do you have athlete's foot, anal irritation or any
  other chronic fungal infections of the skin or nails?

		C	

Count up the number of highlighted A's, G's, C's
and H's

A	G	C	H

A for Allergies

0–5 It is unlikely that you have a major problem with allergies, unless you are already avoiding the substances to which you might be allergic.

6–10 There is a good chance that allergy may be contributing to your current health problems. Read Chapter 16 carefully, and consider avoiding wheat and dairy produce for a trial period of 14 days and seeking guidance from a nutrition consultant.

10 or more There is a strong probability that allergy is contributing to your health problems. Read Chapter 16 carefully, avoid wheat and dairy produce for a trial period of 14 days, and see a nutrition consultant.

G for Glucose Imbalance

0–4 It is unlikely that you have a pronounced glucose imbalance.

5–7 There is a possibility that glucose imbalance may be contributing to your health problems. Read Chapter 15 carefully, avoid all sugar and stimulants for a trial period of 30 days, and consider seeking guidance from a nutrition consultant. Also, make sure your supplement program provides at least 50mg of B1, B2, B5 (pantothenic acid) and B6,

1000mg of vitamin C, 100mcg chromium, 600mg calcium and 400mg magnesium.

8 or more   There is a strong probability that glucose imbalance is contributing to your health problems. Read Chapter 15 carefully, avoid all sugar and stimulants for a trial period of 30 days, and see a nutrition consultant. Also, make sure your supplement program provides at least 50mg of B1, B2, B5 (pantothenic acid) and B6, 1000mg of vitamin C, 100mcg chromium, 600mg calcium and 400mg magnesium.

C for Candida
0–5   It is unlikely that you have candidiasis.

6–14   There is a possibility that you have candidiasis. Read Chapter 17 carefully. If it rings bells you should seek the guidance of a nutrition consultant who can test whether or not you do have candidiasis and, if so, advise you on what to do about it.

15 or more   There is a strong probability you have candidiasis. Read Chapter 17 carefully. The only way to confirm candidiasis is by having a test. We recommend you do this by seeing a nutrition consultant.

H for Hormone Imbalance
0–5   It is unlikely that you have a major hormonal imbalance.

6–14   There is a possibility that you have a degree of hormonal imbalance. You should benefit greatly from applying the advice given throughout this book and by supplementing the correction levels of nutrients given in Chapter 25.

15 or more   There is a strong probability that you have a hormonal imbalance. You should benefit greatly from applying the advice given throughout this book and by supplementing the correction levels of nutrients given in Chapter 25. We also recommend that you seek the guidance of a nutrition consultant who can advise you about the need to test for hormone imbalances and, if there is an imbalance, whether you need to correct it with natural hormone supplements. Natural hormones are only available on prescription. Your nutrition consultant can liaise with your GP or advise a doctor experienced in the use of natural progesterone.

Chapters 8 to 17 deal with specific hormone-related health problems and include advice on which vitamins and minerals to take. In each case, you can find the appropriate maintenance or correction dosage in the chart in Chapter 25.

CHAPTER 8

BEATING PMS WITH DIET

Only in the last two decades has PMS become recognized as a genuine health problem. The symptoms begin during the two weeks prior to a period and usually end an hour to a few days after menstruation starts. Somewhere around half of all menstruating women suffer from PMS, 10 per cent severely. The specific combination of symptoms is very individual, but common ones include anxiety, irritability, fluid retention, mood swings, bloating, breast tenderness, weight gain, acne, fatigue, sweet cravings and forgetfulness.

DIFFERENT TYPES OF PMS

There are several types of PMS that have different symptoms but they often overlap.

PMS Associated with High Estrogen and Low Progesterone Levels

This is the category that 75 per cent of PMS sufferers are said to fall into. A simple saliva test can help identify whether you are estrogen dominant. If you are, you should follow all the recommendations in this book for reducing estrogen levels, including increasing your intake of fiber, ensuring a good intake of phytosterols and B vitamins, eating organically grown produce, limiting exposure to xenoestrogens and reducing consumption of high-fat meat and dairy produce. In a clinical trial, taking B6 in the range of 200–800mg reduced blood estrogen, increased progesterone and reduced symptoms.

According to Dr John Lee, "A surplus of estrogen or a deficiency of progesterone during the two weeks before a period allows an abnormal month-long exposure to estrogen dominance, setting the stage for the symptoms of estrogens side effects," described on page 139. Too much estrogen also increases copper levels; high copper can deplete the body of zinc, and both high copper and low zinc are associated with depression.

Dr John Lee also states that a low thyroid function may simulate the symptoms of PMS. Thyroid hormone activity can be impaired by too much estrogen. Your doctor or nutritionist can recommend and interpret a thyroid function test for you to measure thyroid hormones. For a full screen of thyroid hormones it is advisable to measure T3, T4, TSH and thyroid antibodies.

PMS Associated with Food Cravings

This type of PMS affects about 30 per cent of sufferers. Such women can tolerate increased amounts of carbohydrate foods before symptoms become apparent. They usually have a low level of magnesium in their red blood cells and essential polyunsaturated oils are often deficient. Supplementing magnesium reduces cravings and other symptoms too. Too much refined sugar causes a loss of magnesium and chromium in the urine; supplementing chromium helps control blood glucose levels. Reducing overall carbohydrate intake, particularly refined carbohydrates, is desirable. And including protein with each meal helps to modify the effects of carbohydrates on blood glucose levels. This means eating fish, chicken, nuts, seeds, yoghurt, cheese or pulses with each intake of food. Rice cakes with nut butter would be a good snack.

One of the most potent determinants of appetite is the presence of nutrients in the blood. High-calorie, low-nutrient diets, high in biscuits, cakes and confectionery, may give rise to cravings because the brain never receives the message that the body is nutritionally satisfied despite more than adequate calorific intake. Eating nutritious wholefoods, dense in nutrients, should help control cravings.

PMS Associated with Water Retention

This type of PMS affects between 65 and 75 per cent of sufferers. B6, magnesium and vitamin E have been shown to be helpful. Reducing sodium (salt) intake is also beneficial. Excess sodium increases the likelihood of developing water retention. Many women are prescribed diuretics to help remove the retained water. Diuretics are effective; however, they can deplete the body of potassium and they do not tackle the root cause of the problem.

PMS Associated with High Progesterone Levels

A small percentage of sufferers have higher progesterone levels than normal in the second half of the cycle. They are prone to depression. Vitamin B6, C and magnesium may help.

FACTORS CONTRIBUTING TO PMS

Too Much Stress

Stress is central to the PMS picture. Continued adrenal stimulation often results in nervous tension and anxiety, as described in Chapter 15. Stress depresses the neurotransmitter dopamine involved in mood which may lead to depression. Dopamine is a diuretic, so a deficiency may lead to sodium and water retention. Stress can also raise estrogen levels.

Low Essential Fats

A good intake of essential fats is vital in controlling the symptoms of PMS. It appears that women with PMS are low in these. Eating too much saturated fat inhibits the production of an important prostaglandin called PgE1 (derived from essential fats). Low levels of PgE1 may lead to excessive release of insulin after sugar intake, which decreases blood sugar levels, leading to fatigue and irritability.

A deficiency of essential fats, either from a low intake, poor absorption or impaired conversion to GLA (the essential fat found in abundance in evening primrose, borage or starflower oil), may lead to an apparent excess of the female hormone prolactin, which is involved in mood and water balance.

Low production of PgE1 may contribute to heavy periods. Eating too much saturated fat also promotes the production of less desirable prostaglandins called PgE2 which are involved in inflammatory and clotting mechanisms in the body. (See page 96 which describes more fully dealing with heavy periods.)

Headaches associated with PMS may be partly due to the effect of PgE2 which brings about the clumping of cells (clumping of platelet cells is associated with headaches and migraines). Taking niacin, as described on page 74, when you feel a headache coming on, may help to relieve this symptom. Glucose imbalance, allergies and candidiasis may all give rise to headaches. Check out the relevant chapters and follow the guidelines as appropriate.

A deficiency of the nutrients involved in converting the essential fats into PgE1 may also contribute to the above symptoms. These nutrients include vitamin B6, B3, biotin and C, and the minerals magnesium, zinc and calcium.

Low Magnesium Levels

Low magnesium is associated with poor appetite, nausea, apathy, tiredness, mood changes and muscle cramps. Magnesium is needed at the very first stage of the process in which glucose is converted into energy. Most PMS sufferers have reduced energy levels, and many are deficient in magnesium from nuts, seeds and dark green leafy vegetables. In one study involving 105 women with PMS, 45 per cent had low magnesium levels. PMS often starts after childbirth. Magnesium requirements increase during pregnancy and the growing baby will scavenge what is available, possibly leaving the mother deficient. Low magnesium levels may decrease dopamine levels, contributing to depression; they are also associated with an increase in the hormone aldosterone which can lead to water retention and excess weight gain.

Low B Vitamins

B vitamins are important for the production of energy and stabilizing mood. Low levels of vitamin B1 are associated with a lack of energy, and with anxiety, depression, aggressiveness and poor memory. Vitamin B3 is essential for energy production and sugar balance in the body. Vitamin B5 plays a key role in the production of energy and in keeping the adrenal glands functioning well. Vitamin B6 needs vitamin B2 and the mineral magnesium to work properly. B6 is needed for the production of insulin, so is vital for glucose balance. A low level of vitamin B6 is associated with an excess of estrogen in relation to progesterone. Vitamin B6 was shown to double the amount of magnesium in red blood cells after 100mg of B6 was given twice a day for four weeks. Vitamin

B6 is also needed for choline to function, and choline is needed to clear estrogens from the liver. A complex of B vitamins have been used successfully in PMS, suggesting that syndromes related to estrogen excess are partly caused by the liver failing to inactivate estrogen because of a deficiency of B vitamins.

Too Much Alcohol

Alcohol intake can contribute to the symptoms of PMS by upsetting glucose balance, and by inhibiting the absorption and/or use of essential nutrients like magnesium, zinc and some B vitamins.

PMS is a complex syndrome and the approach to its management has to be multifaceted. If simple measures fail to bring relief, working with a nutritionist is the best policy. Follow the Diet for the Good Life (Chapter 23) as a starting point, then the advice in Beating the Sugar Blues (Chapter 15), The Allergy Connection (Chapter 16) and Conquering Candida (Chapter 17). Supplementing a basic level of nutrients plus essential oils should be part of the initial program.

CHAPTER 9

FERTILITY RIGHTS AND WRONGS

Infertility has been recorded since ancient times – the Bible makes references to the "barren" woman. Throughout history, infertility has somehow been seen as a punishment and the barren woman has often been portrayed as bitter and somehow responsible for her own condition. It is only relatively recently that we have realized that up to 40 per cent of infertility problems relate to the man and around 80 per cent of birth defects are the result of damaged sperm. Around one in four couples have fertility problems. Even for those who don't, it is not uncommon for successful conception to take between six and 18 months.

THE CAUSES OF INFERTILITY

In women, blocked fallopian tubes are a common cause of infertility, most frequently arising after abdominal surgery because of scarring and adhesions. Gynecological problems, such as pelvic inflammatory disease, endometriosis and infections, can also contribute to blocked fallopian tubes and infertility. Infections can contribute to this problem. Excess acidity of the cervical mucus is also associated with infertility, as it creates an environment that is hostile to sperm from the moment they enter the vagina. Improving your diet, with particular emphasis on increasing your intake of alkaline-forming foods (see Chapter 23), helps normalize excess acidity in the body.

Being underweight is associated with difficulty in becoming pregnant, with absence of periods or anovulatory cycles being a major cause of infertility. In earlier centuries, when a woman was producing offspring in times of fluctuating food supplies, it was important for her to carry on her body all the energy required – stored as fat – to complete the growth of the developing baby, even if food supplies ran short. To maintain regular periods and fertility, it appears that about 22 per cent body fat is required. Loss of periods is not uncommon in young women athletes who have a hard training schedule. If trying to conceive it would be sensible to change to a less demanding regime. Similarly, women with anorexia nervosa often have no periods.

New research is also indicating that those women who do not regularly ovulate and are also overweight are as much, if not more, at risk of infertility as underweight women. Maintaining an ideal body weight should increase the chances of becoming pregnant.

INFERTILITY PROGRAMS

In the twentieth century, we have discovered ingenious ways of helping infertile couples have babies. The technique of in vitro fertilization (IVF) has already transformed the lives of many childless couples. This is the technique whereby an ovum is fertilized by a sperm outside the body and then replaced in the uterus. IVF pregnancies are usually supported by heavy doses of synthetic hormones.

However, before embarking on complicated, potentially toxic, hormonal programs to increase fertility, you should give your body the best chance to conceive naturally, particularly when you have no known, specific condition that is affecting your fertility. Even if you do have such a condition, good nutrition should help support the success of an artificially engineered pregnancy. If you are being advised to go on a hormonal program due to your partner's low sperm count, encourage your partner to seek a nutritionist to identify nutritional deficiencies and to embark on an optimum nutrition program. Ideally, a preconceptual care program would be for a minimum of three months, preferably six, for both partners. The long-term health of babies born under the influence of high-level synthetic hormones has yet to be fully researched. A nutritionist can work with you to optimize your diet and help identify, through testing, any nutritional imbalances or other factors that may be affecting your ability to conceive. Several ION-trained nutritionists specialize in preconceptual care and can be contacted through Foresight, an organization committed to helping couples increase their chances of conception and having a healthy baby.

FERTILITY WRONGS

As part of an overall program to maximize your chances of conception – good nutrition and little stress – there are also several factors to avoid. Many are described in detail in the next chapter, such as not conceiving if you have recently had an infection or have candidiasis (see also Chapter 17), weight loss and others. Obvious substances to avoid are alcohol, cigarettes and non-prescription drugs. It is also wise to avoid supplementing more than 7500iu of vitamin A daily in the form of retinol (beta-carotene is not known to be toxic), as it is associated with fetal abnormalities.

SYNTHETIC HORMONES

Many women have spent years on the Pill, a method of contraception that works by preventing ovulation. One in every

200 women's periods will cease after stopping the Pill, but fertility will return in most cases within two years.

As part of an infertility program, many women are treated with drugs to stimulate ovulation, even when they are shown to be ovulating spontaneously. These are often the same women who have previously taken the Pill. What is often not considered as part of most infertility treatments is that natural hormone production and hormone receptor sites within the cells need a good supply of zinc and magnesium to work effectively, and these vital minerals are both depleted by the Pill.

The use of synthetic hormones before and during pregnancy, and through lactation, exposes a baby at its most critical stages of development. This is the time when sex, intelligence and future health are being determined. It is known that hormones taken by the mother in early pregnancy can cause cancer and genital abnormalities in her children.[1] The results of a study involving 5700 pregnancies showed a remarkably low incidence of congenital abnormalities in children born to women who had never taken the Pill, compared to women who had regularly taken it.[2]

Depo-provera and Noristerat are injectable progestogens (synthetic forms of progesterone). Provera carries the warning that its use in early pregnancy may increase the risk of early abortion or congenital deformities of the fetus. In order to give the body a chance to restore its natural hormone balance, women are generally advised to wait at least three months before attempting to get pregnant once they have stopped using the contraceptive pill. We recommend that you wait at least six months to allow the synthetic hormones to be fully eliminated from the body.

NATURAL FAMILY PLANNING

Pregnancy will occur only if a viable sperm meets an egg. The egg only survives for up to 24 hours after release, whereas the sperm can survive for three to six days. It is therefore important to capture this period of time to maximize the chances of conception. Given that many cycles do not fit into the classic 28 days, it can be difficult to know when you have ovulated. However, there is a simple method that can help you identify this, and there are natural family planning teachers available to help you understand what you need to do. Essentially, the method involves three steps:

- **Checking cervical mucus:** With increasing estrogen levels, the cervical mucus changes at ovulation from being cloudy, thick and sticky to a more watery, clear and slippery fluid. It also becomes alkaline, which sperm like.

- **Checking the cervix:** Changes occur in the cervix in synchrony with the changes in the cervical mucus. When the egg is about to be fertilized, the mouth of the cervix opens, to enable the sperm to meet the egg. Otherwise the mouth of the cervix remains closed. These changes can be felt.

- **Checking the temperature:** The rise of progesterone just after ovulation increases body temperature by at least 0.2 degrees centigrade. This is a simple test that many women use to identify whether they have ovulated. In an average four-week cycle, ovulation usually takes place on day 14. By taking your temperature each day and recording it on a graph, you can easily tell when you have ovulated because your temperature will rise by at least 0.2 degrees centigrade. For those with longer, shorter or irregular cycles, the graph is a useful means of identifying when ovulation has occurred.

The success of this natural method depends on the motivation of the woman wishing to become pregnant and how well she has been taught. Some women do find it difficult to identify the different states of the cervical mucus, although one researcher found that 97 per cent of women could do so,[3] and others find the process of self-examination unpleasant.

Ovulation predictor kits, which are also useful, are now available in large drug stores. Both the natural method and predictor kits can be used to avoid pregnancy, as well as to enhance the chances of becoming pregnant.

The following chapter explains more fully how to use a natural approach to maximize your chances of conceiving, maintaining a healthy pregnancy, and having a healthy baby.

CHAPTER 10

···

MAKING HEALTHY BABIES

What a parent eats before and, in the case of the mother, during, pregnancy is very significant for the health of a baby. All nutrients are essential for fertility, and, by definition, all are needed for proper development. Yet, even so-called well-balanced diets fall short of recommended intakes of specific nutrients. Whatever foods are chosen, the body will do its utmost to perform optimally – that is the way it is designed. Yet it is virtually impossible to achieve optimum nutrition from low-quality foods. So there is no more important time to aim for the best nutrition than when preparing for a pregnancy.

According to Professor Michael Crawford, Professor of Nutrition and Biochemistry at Queen Elizabeth's Hospital for Children, nutrition not only determines individual health, but has shaped the development of our species. In his co-authored book *The Driving Force* he describes nutrition as the factor that has driven the evolutionary process. He reasons that humans developed into such a highly complex species because part of our evolution was at the seashore. The human brain and nervous system are composed primarily of polyunsaturated oil (unlike most animals who contain largely saturated fats). Polyunsaturated oils are liquid, which allows very rapid nerve transmissions that enable humans to perform very complex tasks. The sea is a rich source of polyunsaturated oils from its vegetation and fish.

THE FATS OF LIFE

The human heart and blood vessels are also rich in polyunsaturated oils. Both the nervous system and cardiovascular systems form very early in embryonic life, the first three months of pregnancy. They are both primitive systems from which we have evolved. Many of the degenerative diseases we see today attack the nerves and blood vessels. Polyunsaturated oils have widespread effects in the body, including helping to regulate immunity and hormones. Polyunsaturated oils are vital for healthy sperm, and the control of the female reproductive cycle.

Ensuring a sufficient intake of polyunsaturated oil in a form that is healthy for the body is crucial for human development. Good sources are fresh nuts and seeds and their oils, wholegrains and fish. Polyunsaturated oils are very delicate and need to be handled with care; they are easily damaged when heated, making them harmful to the body. Nuts and seeds are best eaten raw and oils are best used for salad dressings, in fruit shakes or vegetable juices, and instead of butter on jacket potatoes. Special oils, called Omega 3 oils, found in flax seed (linseed), walnut and soya oils and fish, have been researched and shown to have beneficial effects on reproduction. Omega 3 oils are deficient in the average diet.

A CASE FOR PRECONCEPTUAL CARE

The importance of this cannot be overstated. In the modern world we are exposed to a plethora of previously unknown harmful agents from our environment and our food, the effects of which are only just beginning to be realized. With knowledge, however, we can choose to avoid some of these, and eat healthy, wholesome food. Boosting the body's resistance to the environment is a strong and positive way of increasing the chances of having a healthy baby who can mature into a healthy adult.

The most serious threats to a potential new life arise during the development of the egg and sperm, and then during the first three months of development in the uterus. Sperm take about four months to mature and the egg about one month. So prospective fathers need to be health-conscious for at least four months before conception. For women, the most critical time is one month before conception, and the first three months of pregnancy, when the differentiation of organs and limbs is determined.

Smoking and Alcohol

Many pregnancies are unplanned; many others happen under the influence of alcohol, medications and nicotine. According to the detailed research of Arthur and Margaret Wynne, published in their book, *The Case for Preconception Care of Men and Women*, alcohol and nicotine are likely to have their most damaging effects at the time of conception and immediately following conception. While most of their evidence is based on animal research, they propose that humans are likely to respond similarly. Many women only make the decision to avoid alcohol and smoking once they know they are pregnant, which is usually around six to eight weeks after conception.

Around one in four pregnancies are estimated to end in a miscarriage and the real figure is likely to be higher, as many miscarriages go unreported. Some experts believe that miscarriage is a sensitive indicator that the parents are exposed to environmental hazards. One study found that the mother drinking alcohol daily, even in moderation, increased the risk of miscarriage[4]. There is no safe limit for smoking or alcohol during pregnancy. The most dangerous time is soon after conception when the cells are rapidly dividing. The worst-case scenario of alcohol in pregnancy is a baby born with fetal alcohol syndrome which is recognized by low birth weight, mild facial deformities and a high predisposition towards ear infections, squints, congenital hip deformities, fused digits and deafness.

Nutritional and Other Factors

Deficiencies of essential polyunsaturated oils, zinc, manganese and vitamin E are associated with recurrent miscarriages. Other causes of miscarriage include diabetes and thyroid problems.

Caffeine has also been shown to adversely affect reproduction in men and women.

Infections

Infections such as cytomegalovirus, chlamydia and herpes can all cause miscarriages.

We recommend that you avoid conceiving at a point when you know that you have an infection or have recently been exposed to an infection. Infections from a variety of sources, including rubella, mumps, chicken pox, cytomegalovirus, lysteria and toxoplasmosis, have all been associated with fertility problems and/or the baby being born with abnormalities. Candida albicans is a yeast organism which commonly becomes fungal in nature (see Chapter 17). We recommend a full screen for genito-urinary infections before you start trying to conceive.

Libido

It goes without saying that having a desire for sex will increase the chances of pregnancy. Reduced libido affects both men and women and can be worsened by a variety of factors, including psychological, hormonal, disease, surgery, stress, drugs, alcohol and high exposure to heavy metals. The physiological and hormonal changes that accompany stress and depression may contribute to low sexual interest by affecting the central nervous system and creating a reduction in testosterone, which is required for sexual desire. Several studies show a significant and consistent depression of blood testosterone levels in men under stress. Studies are also being undertaken to evaluate the effects of smoking on testosterone levels. One study showed reduced glucose tolerance in a group of men who had become impotent, having previously had normal sexual functioning.

Health of Sperm

The average sperm count has dropped by 50 per cent in the last 50 years. Low sperm counts are associated with exposure to hormone-disrupting chemicals, testosterone deficiency and a poor diet. The head of the sperm is rich in the amino acid arginine and the mineral zinc. Supplementing both zinc and arginine has been shown to raise sperm count in infertile men. Zinc and magnesium deficiency are associated with abnormal sperm shape and motility. Zinc is needed at every stage of the reproductive process in both men and women. In the developing fetus, zinc is required to help trigger the gene that differentiates cells into the "right" cells, such as skin, brain or nerve cells. The average man takes in 7.6mg of zinc a day, and up to 3mg can be lost per ejaculation. Infertile men tend to have low zinc levels; and men given a zinc-deficient diet show decreased sperm counts and testosterone levels.

In one study, 37 men with a history of infertility for seven years or more were given the equivalent of 36mg of zinc. Results showed that those with normal testosterone levels had no significant changes in sperm count, but 22 of the men who had low testosterone levels to start with, had increased sperm counts and testosterone after zinc supplementation. Nine men later went on to father a child.

Both high and low levels of the mineral selenium are likely to be problematic. Too little is associated with a low sperm count, abnormally shaped sperm and non-viable sperm. In animal studies a lack of selenium induced damaged sperm. Too much selenium can be toxic. Vitamin A, also, is needed for normal sperm shape. One group of researchers found that when 87 men were given 50,000iu of retinol (a form of vitamin A) a day, over half of them had increased sperm counts and healthier sperm.[5] Ideal intake is around 10,000iu. When vitamin B12 was given to two infertile men over a period of seven months their sperm count increased from three to 32 million per milliliter, and the mobility and health of their sperm greatly improved.

Sometimes normal sperm count and sperm function may not be enough for fertilization. Fifteen male volunteers who had low fertilization rates in attempts at in vitro fertilization (IVF) were given 300iu of vitamin E per day.[6] The success rate increased from 10 to 29 per cent within one month of treatment. The researchers suggest that the antioxidant activity of vitamin E may enhance sperm's fertilization potential.

Although nutrient deficiencies are linked to reduced sperm counts, the most potent factor is the toxic chemicals that end up in our water supplies as end products of the chemical and plastics industries. As described in Part 2, these chemicals and pesticides have the ability to mimic estrogen in the body. Estrogen is a female hormone, of which men have just a little in their bodies naturally. This excessive exposure to estrogen has been shown to bring about reproductive changes in fish. For this reason, although fish are a rich source of polyunsaturated oils, we recommend that fish are avoided at this critical time due to their high toxic exposure. Rely instead on flax seed, walnut and soya oil for the Omega 3 oils or a guaranteed PCB-free supplement of eicosapentaenoic acid (EPA). Bags of potato chips and other similarly packaged fatty foods are also best avoided because fatty foods can absorb estrogenic-like chemicals from the plastic packaging. You can greatly reduce your exposure to environmental estrogens by eating organic food and avoiding fatty foods packaged or stored in plastic. Many foods, including soya, wheat, citrus, fennel and alfalfa, contain natural estrogen-like substances which are thought to be beneficial.

Health of Eggs

Adequate protein intake is an absolute must for egg production. Animal studies show that insufficient protein results in a reduced number of eggs, and if conception occurs it is associated with a high number of embryonic deaths. Around 60g of protein a day is recommended for conception by Margaret and Arthur Wynne. Vegetable protein is a good source and far less hazardous than animal protein. Animal proteins, when cooked at temperatures above 150 degrees centigrade, can damage the genetic material of the egg. These temperatures are often exceeded in cooking, especially frying. The nitroso compounds used to preserve ham, bacon, preserved meats, some cheeses and smoked products are also capable of damaging the genetic material of the egg in animal studies.

B vitamins are crucial for fertility and the early development of the embryo. Animal studies have shown that a lack of vitamin B1 can inhibit the release of the egg, impede the implantation of the egg in the uterus and bring about malformations.[7] Both vitamin B2 and B6 deficiency are associated with sterility in animal studies. Vitamin B12 and folic acid deficiency slows down the production of DNA, the blueprint of our genetic material, and RNA, the messenger that transcribes the genetic code used to carry out the cell's instruction. B12 and folic acid deficiency have been shown to damage chromosomes, the individual sections making up the genetic codes. Folic acid deficiency is now unequivocally linked to neural tube defects in humans.

B vitamins are vital for hormonal control. When they are deficient the endocrine system recognizes the inadequacy and shuts down the reproductive process. This is considered to be an evolutionary design to protect against abnormalities. However, sub-optimum nutrition does not necessarily close down the reproductive processes and may increase the chances of a less than healthy pregnancy continuing.

Zinc, magnesium and vitamin A are vital for egg production, and zinc is vital for the growth and development of the embryo. As many as 97 per cent of couples referred for preconceptual care show evidence of zinc deficiency. Heavy metals like lead and cadmium impair zinc use and can interfere with the development of the baby's nervous system.

A HEALTHY PREGNANCY

It is most important for the mother to keep healthy during pregnancy. The hormone progesterone – a "quietening" hormone – is produced in very large amounts during this time. We are led to believe that pregnant women should be bordering on the bionic: coping with the stresses of pregnancy, work and a family. But it is natural to slow down and feel tired, particularly during the first few months. This may be nature's way of ensuring the survival of the young embryo.

Sometimes insufficient progesterone is produced to maintain pregnancy, a known cause of early miscarriage. This can be linked to stress, so resting in this early stage of pregnancy, particularly if you have had a history of early miscarriage, is essential. If you have a miscarriage, we recommend that you have your saliva hormone levels tested by a nutritionist for estrogen and progesterone on day 21 of a normal 28-day cycle. Supplementing a natural source of progesterone under the guidance of your medical practitioner, as described in Part 4, is worth considering if progesterone production is found to be low. A nutritionist would be able to work with you and recommend appropriate tests.

A good wholefood diet appears to ease the minor ailments associated with pregnancy. Drink at least 600ml (1 pint) good-quality water daily, alongside a diet high in fruit and vegetables, to help combat urine infections which are more easily contracted during pregnancy. If you have (or suspect you have) any allergies to food, then pregnancy is a good time to identify them. There is accumulating data to show that avoiding food allergens in pregnancy and during breastfeeding can help prevent the baby developing these allergies too. Common food allergens are to wheat and dairy produce.

Eating a wide and diverse diet on a daily basis maximizes potential for optimal nutrient intake from food. Ensure that you have a range of grains in your diet, including rye, oats, barley, rice, corn, millet, buckwheat and quinoa. Most good healthfood stores stock a variety of products using these grains, including flakes which make good muesli, flours for baking and pastas. Reduce dairy produce; nuts, seeds and green leafy vegetables supply excellent levels of calcium and magnesium (whereas dairy produce is only rich in calcium) and both are needed. Selecting from beans, lentils, nuts, seeds, wholegrains, a little fish if desired, chicken and free-range eggs on a daily basis at each meal will ensure that you receive enough protein.

A study involving 5000 Hungarian women taking a multi-vitamin and mineral containing 800mcg of folic acid, compared to a control group, showed fewer per cent congenital malformations in the supplemented group.[8] Studies also show that most women are not consuming the recommended intakes for specific vitamins and minerals. Food intake in pregnancy increases by 15–20 per cent. The requirements for folic acid, vitamin B, C, calcium, zinc and magnesium increase by 30–100 per cent. It is important that a mother chooses foods that are rich in nutrients, and not simply high in calories. Even the best of diets does not provide the correct levels of all the nutrients needed for pregnancy. Folic acid has now been confirmed as essential in preventing spina bifida. It is therefore wise to take a specially prepared pregnancy formula that has been designed to meet both the needs of the mother and her developing baby. Key nutrients to supplement during pregnancy are vitamin B12 and B6, folic acid, zinc and iron.

However, care must be taken with supplements: we recommend that you seek expert help to formulate your individual supplementary needs preconceptually and during pregnancy.

Recommended Safe Supplement Intake for Pregnancy

Supplement	Quantity	Supplier
Prenatal Supplements	2 a day	Solgar
Calcium and magnesium citrate	3 a day	Solgar
Omega 3 Oils	2 tablespoons a day with food	Flora
or Essential Balance	2 tablespoons a day	Omega Nutrition

MANAGING COMMON AILMENTS OF PREGNANCY

Morning Sickness

In our experience, morning sickness is relieved by changing to the Diet for the Good Life (see Chapter 23). Dealing with stress and food cravings, and following a diet to balance blood glucose levels, helps many women. Morning sickness usually stops around the twelfth or fourteenth week of pregnancy. If it persists beyond this, you should seek medical advice. Morning sickness has been shown to respond well to 50mg of vitamin B6 twice a day, and 200–500mg of magnesium once a day, plus sufficient B12 and folic acid.

Cravings

Low zinc levels are associated with the abnormal cravings a woman often experiences in early pregnancy. In addition, replenishing low iron levels in the body has been successfully used to control the abnormal cravings that some women experience for strange, and sometimes harmful, substances, such as chalk or coal.

Constipation and Varicose Veins

These often occur together and are common in pregnancy due to changes in hormone levels, which make the muscles more relaxed. A good wholefood diet, containing plenty of fiber, is beneficial. Some women who develop varicose veins have been shown to be low in vitamin B6.

Pre-eclampsia

Studies have shown that women who took a daily 10mg supplement of vitamin B6 had a significantly lower incidence of pre-eclampsia (toxemia of pregnancy), than those who did not.[9] Pre-eclampsia is recognized by water retention, weight gain, increasing blood pressure, and the appearance of protein in the urine. Low levels of zinc have also been found in women with pre-eclampsia.

Blood Pressure

Raised blood pressure commonly occurs in pregnancy and an optimum diet should help to control it. Evening primrose oil and calcium have both been successfully used to reduce it.

Heartburn

Many antacids commonly taken for heartburn contain aluminium which some evidence has shown to be toxic. A quarter of a teaspoonful of sodium bicarbonate dissolved in water and taken between meals can bring relief, but a change of diet is a priority. Eating five times a day – three small meals and two snacks, including plenty of wholefoods and fruits and vegetables – should help alleviate heartburn.

A SUCCESSFUL LABOR

Stock up on complex carbohydrates during the last two weeks of pregnancy. This means eating plenty of wholegrains and vegetables. Complex carbohydrates are the main energy source for the body. It is still the practice in some hospitals to starve women in labor just in case there is a need for an anesthetic. However, in terms of energy requirements, labor can be compared to a marathon run. After all the good work you have done to create a healthy baby, the last thing you want is to run out of energy, have a prolonged labor that may result in a cesarean section, deprive yourself of a natural birth and increase your baby's risks of birth-related trauma. If your hospital allows you to eat and drink, we recommend that you drink diluted grape juice, a very healthy and readily available source of fruit sugar that should help keep up your energy levels. Tea containing stimulants may not give you stable energy levels.

A HEALTHY BABY

Having put all your effort into achieving a healthy baby, you now have an 18-year commitment to helping this new life achieve optimum health. This means continuing your healthy diet and lifestyle in the long term. The father's responsibility does not stop the moment he knows his partner is pregnant. Raising a healthy family is a full-time, on-going commitment.

The wisest thing any unborn child can do is to choose parents who took their health seriously before conception! In this way, the human species can look forward to optimum health, based on knowledge and responsibility, in the generations to come.

CHAPTER 11

Secrets for a Trouble-free Menopause

The menopause should occur gradually, allowing the body to adapt to the changes with ease. For many women, it is not the fear of osteoporosis, breast cancer or heart disease that most concerns them but how to cope with the debilitating symptoms that affect their daily lives – hot flashes, vaginal dryness, joint pains, insomnia, headaches and depression. The usual remedy prescribed by doctors is HRT. Rarely are women educated about how they can help themselves to cope with the menopause naturally, so let's take a look at a natural approach to some of the most problematic symptoms.

Hot Flashes

Three-quarters of menopausal women, particularly those who are thin, experience some hot flashes. These are not directly a sign of estrogen deficiency, but a result of increased activity of the hypothalamus gland in the brain to bring about the production of follicle stimulating hormone (FSH) and luteinizing hormone (LH). Extra-high levels of these two hormones occur as the menopause approaches, in an attempt to stimulate any remaining eggs to develop. Meanwhile, estrogen levels fall, ovulation becomes infrequent and progesterone levels decline rapidly. Giving natural progesterone, usually in the form of a cream rubbed on the skin, reduces hot flashes, probably by increasing receptors in hormone-sensitive cells.

Hot flashes may also be reduced by supplementing vitamin E, vitamin C and bioflavonoids. When vitamin E levels are low, there is a tendency for FSH and LH to increase. Vitamin E also appears to stabilise hormone levels.

Sexual Problems

A lack of sex drive can result from a variety of reasons, not all nutritional. Chapter 10 discusses some of the other possible causes. Good nutrition may make you feel better, in turn increasing your sexual desire. If not, you may wish to contact a sex therapist or counsellor.

Vaginal dryness is another reason for declining interest in sex. The vagina is kept moist because it produces vaginal secretions but declining estrogen levels tend to dry up these secretions. However, the adrenal glands continue to produce estrogens, as do fat cells, during and after the menopause. Vitamin E cream used locally has helped many women with vaginitis. Supplementing vitamins A and C, plus zinc, are also important for keeping vaginal membranes healthy.

Natural estrogen creams, in the form of estriol, have been successful in treating vaginitis and can also reduce the occurrence of urinary tract infections, restore normal vaginal mucous membranes, and provide the right environment in the vagina to inhibits the growth of unfriendly organisms. Dr Lee found that, when these women used progesterone creams rubbed into the skin to treat their vaginitis, they experienced similar benefits to those using estrogen cream. Progesterone cream is preferable for women who are advised against using estrogen therapy because of a history of breast, ovarian or uterine cancer.

Insomnia

Women the world over sleep less as they get older, which may be a protective mechanism so that the young are protected by their elders in the small hours. So long as the sleep you experience is refreshing, it's best to get up and do something productive and enjoy the peace, rather than worry about not sleeping. For those of you who like to meditate, the early hours of the morning are reputed to be the best time and meditation can compensate for sleep.

Stimulants, such as caffeine in tea and coffee and nicotine in cigarettes, can disrupt sleeping patterns and are best avoided. Caffeine also acts as a diuretic, causing frequent visits to the bathroom during the night. Camomile or lime blossom tea are relaxants. So too are the minerals calcium and magnesium, plentiful in green, leafy vegetables, nuts and seeds.

Headaches

Some headaches are caused by blood vessels in the head narrowing, possibly as a result of declining estrogen levels, since estrogen dilates blood vessels, improving blood flow. Vitamin B3 (as niacin) helps widen blood vessels and can be taken preventatively, in a 100mg dose, if you feel a headache coming on. This form of vitamin B3 can cause a temporary hot flashing sensation as it widens blood vessels (in this way it helps to alleviate headaches). Coffee, alcohol and red wine frequently give rise to headaches, as can a food allergy, candidiasis, or glucose imbalance.

Joint Pains

Vitamin B6 supplementation has been shown to help painful nodules on finger joints if treated early. Vitamin B6, like all B vitamins, is best taken as part of a B complex. Food intolerance may manifest at the menopause and may contribute to joint pains. Wheat and dairy produce are the common offenders (see Chapter 16). The essential fats GLA and EPA have potent anti-inflammatory properties and can help reduce the inflammation that contributes to joint pain. Vitamin B6, B3, biotin and vitamin C, plus the minerals zinc, calcium and magnesium, all play an important role in helping essential fats create anti-inflammatory prostaglandins. Too much red meat and full-fat dairy produce help to create a type of prostaglandin that increases inflammation in the body.

Dr John Lee, and other doctors have found that many of their patients have gained relief from chronic aches and pains by using natural progesterone, which has anti-inflammatory properties. You can rub progesterone cream or oil directly on the joint or tissue that hurts.

Memory Loss

Research has shown that supplementing vitamin B5 and choline is beneficial during the menopause for the production of acetylcholine, a neurotransmitter needed for memory. Essential fats and phospholipids are vital for maintaining memory. This means eating seeds and nuts or their oils on a regular basis. If this is a problem area you could also consider supplementing phosphatidyl serine 300mg, available in healthfood stores.

Depression

The causes of depression are many, and some of them can be helped by nutrition. Causes can include B vitamin deficiency, stress, imbalance between calcium and magnesium, allergies, candidiasis, or imbalance between estrogens and progesterone. Our mood is very dependent on the foods we eat. Protein foods are broken down to make neurotransmitters, the brain chemicals whose balance very much controls our mood. And protein breaks down to form amino acids and amines. Cheese, red wine and chocolate contain high levels of amines which can exert a powerful, stimulating, and often immediate effect on the brain. If high levels of amines are not broken down, or if the amines are stimulated, depression can follow. Enzymes that break amines down, require zinc, magnesium and B vitamins. When supplemented, these nutrients can relieve depression.

Both zinc and copper play an important role in the brain and their balance is crucial. Too much estrogen can bind copper in the blood and prevent it reaching the brain cells; it also increases the tendency for the blood to clot, which can reduce the oxygen supply to the brain. In addition, it can interact with thyroid hormone by slowing down the metabolism of brain cells. Vitamin E and progesterone enhance cell oxygenation. According to Dr John Lee, many elderly women with signs of senility are likely to gain increased mental acuity as a result of using progesterone. He finds that, when anovulatory pre-menopausal or post-menopausal women take progesterone supplements, their mental clarity and concentration improve.

Heart Disease

Heart disease is the leading cause of death in post-menopausal women. One of the most hailed benefits of taking HRT is that it is said to reduce the risk of developing coronary artery disease after the menopause. (Estrogen levels decline after the menopause, and estrogens are thought to protect blood vessels and blood fat levels.)

This supposed benefit is based on research which showed that women taking HRT had half the risk of developing heart disease, and were less likely to die from that cause than the population as a whole. However, this claim does not stand up to close examination. Research also indicates that women who take estrogens after the menopause are more likely to be upper-middle-class, non-smokers, better educated and better fed – all factors that automatically carry a lower risk for developing heart disease. A UK review in 1991 concluded that evidence of HRT protecting against heart disease is weak or non-existent.[10] Some studies conducted on women taking estrogen-only HRT even suggest that using HRT actually increases the risk of developing heart disease. While estrogens are understood to be beneficial for the blood vessels, it remains unclear whether the ability of estrogens to relax arteries is particularly significant in treating coronary artery disease.

Progestogens were added to HRT preparations to minimize the risk of developing cancer of the lining of the uterus, but these reduce some of the beneficial effects of estrogens on blood fat levels. The potential protection from coronary artery disease is therefore lost when progestogens are added to the HRT. Natural progesterone is, however, beneficial to the cardiovascular system. A study in 1989 found that, when women were given a combination of estrogens and progesterone, their blood fat levels improved. More recently, in 1997, a study on rhesus monkeys, comparing a synthetic progestogen with progesterone, found that the latter was protective against coronary vasospasm.[11]

Raised Blood Pressure

The effect of synthetic estrogens and progestogens on blood pressure is not currently fully realized. These synthetic hormones can cause the body to retain salt and water in the cells, which can ultimately raise blood pressure. When progestogens are combined with estrogens there is an increased risk of developing high blood pressure, whereas natural progesterone helps rid the body of excess sodium (salt), thus lowering blood pressure and water retention.

Synthetic hormones potentially block the natural ability of the body to use beneficial substances that help keep the blood thin. Women taking oral contraceptives or HRT are more likely to have sticky blood and develop blood clots. Thick blood is also a risk factor for high blood pressure and for developing coronary artery disease.

CHAPTER 12

PREVENTING AND REVERSING OSTEOPOROSIS

Osteoporosis is the silent thief that robs your skeleton of up to 25 per cent of its bone mass by the time you reach 50. It is now a serious epidemic in Britain. Bones become porous, or osteoporotic, due to progressive loss of minerals, mass and density which can result in fractures. Every three minutes someone in the UK has a fracture due to osteoporosis: one in three women and one in 12 men have a fracture by the age of 70. Hip fractures ruin 60,000 lives each year, causing severe pain and 15,000 deaths. As much as £750 million is spent each year dealing with the problem and nearly one-third of orthopedic beds are filled by patients with the condition.

Yet skeletal material dating from between 1729 and 1852, unearthed during the restoration of Christ Church, Spitalfields, in London, showed significantly less bone loss in women then than now, despite our supposedly better diet. Investigators found no sign of menopausal change in the unearthed bones. This suggests that some aspect of modern living doesn't suit our skeletons.

FEMININE FRAILTY

Women are more at risk than men of developing osteoporosis. The female hormones estrogen and progesterone are protective of women's bones, just as the male hormone testosterone is protective of men's. But, from the age of 35, women regularly fail to ovulate, minimizing their production of progesterone, the major hormone for bone strength. Women at most risk of developing osteoporosis are those who have had an early menopause (before the age of 45), either naturally, or surgically, by removing the uterus and one or both ovaries.

Major Well-Known Risk Factors in Osteoporosis

- Early menopause
- Anorexia
- Bulimia
- Over-dieted
- Over/under-exercised
- Many missed periods

- Previous fracture from slight injury
- Significant corticosteroid use
- Lost several inches in height
- Close relatives with brittle bones
- Heavy intake of alcohol
- History of heavy cigarette smoking

The two most common treatments for osteoporosis are hormone replacement therapy (HRT) and replenishing the bones with calcium through supplementation. Both methods of treatment have a sound basis. They are, however, simplistic approaches to a complex health problem.

THE ESTROGEN MYTH

Estrogen is, without doubt, important for bone health, but its role has been exaggerated. Women are advised to undergo HRT in the belief that estrogen will protect them from osteoporosis. (Women with a uterus are given a synthetic progestogen to minimize the side-effects of estrogen, particularly the risk of uterine and breast cancer.) Those without a uterus are recommended estrogen-only HRT, but this does not protect their breasts. Estrogen's main role in protecting bones is to stimulate osteoclast cells to clear out old bone, making spaces available for new bone to be laid down in. It is not currently thought to have a direct bone-building action.

However, raising their estrogen levels causes other problems, increasing the imbalance in their hormones. From the age of 35 onwards, women are naturally exposed to higher levels of estrogen than progesterone, as they regularly do not ovulate. Furthermore, progesterone, the bone-building hormone, is only produced in significant amounts after ovulation, whereas estrogen is produced in varying amounts throughout the menstrual cycle.

Osteoporosis is a slow, progressive disease: bone loss starts in most women in their mid-thirties. It does not happen overnight with the last menstrual period; it develops alongside high estrogen levels. Specific bone cells, known as osteoblasts, have receptor sites for progesterone, the main hormone that ensures that new bone is built. Women taking combined HRT do not experience much benefit from the synthetic form of progesterone, as it has only a marginal effect on bone mineral density. There is no conclusive evidence that HRT will protect bones from the ravages of osteoporosis.

THE DRAWBACKS OF HRT

The *New England Journal of Medicine* reported in October 1993 the latest results of an ongoing study of women in Framingham, Massachusetts, USA,[12] saying, "It shows that HRT fails to protect women from osteoporosis – therefore eliminating at a stroke one of the main reasons for its use."

One study researching 670 women, of whom nearly a third were taking estrogen therapy, found that bone mass was only preserved in those women who had taken the therapy for seven years or more.[13] As only 7 per cent of women take HRT for more than eight years, it offers little protection against osteoporosis.

More startling is the fact that even women who have taken HRT for ten years are still not protected from fractures caused by osteoporosis. When such women stopped taking HRT, they had a rapid decline in bone mineral density. By the age of 75, their bone mineral density was found to be only just over 3 per cent higher than in women who had never taken HRT. So, unless you are prepared to take HRT for life, it is unlikely to protect you against osteoporosis, and the longer you take HRT, the greater your risk of developing breast and endometrial cancer.

Thick, sticky blood may also complicate bone formation. Dr Kitty Little, from Oxford, found masses of tiny clots in the bones of rabbits treated with hormones. She is convinced that HRT in the form of estrogen and progestogens increases the risk of osteoporosis. She believes that blood clots in the bones can cause bone to break down, leading to osteoporosis.

IS PROGESTERONE AN ANSWER?

On the other hand, natural progesterone has been shown to improve bone mineral density in women, irrespective of age, when applied topically as a cream – in the required amounts and in a form identical to that produced in the body. Dr John Lee reported in *The Lancet* in 1990 improvements of 15 per cent on average over a three-year period.[14] Dr Lee has been using natural progesterone with his patients for the last 20 years with excellent results and no known serious side-effects. As natural progesterone is a natural substance, it is not patentable, which prevents vast profits being made through its sale. Synthetic hormones, in contrast, *are* patentable, allowing large profits to be made. Certain plant foods contain phyto-chemicals which act like hormones: cultures whose diets are rich in soya and/or wild yam, which both contain such phy-tochemicals, show little evidence of osteoporosis. (For more on phytonutrients, see Chapter 24.)

THE CALCIUM QUESTION

A total of 99 per cent of all the calcium in the body should be in the bones. Only 1 per cent is needed in the blood to ensure that important physical reactions can occur. It may be very convincing for the Milk Marketing Board to suggest that osteoporosis is a calcium problem (as milk is a very rich source of calcium) but your bones do not see it so simplistically. Harvard Medical School researchers have reported that drinking lots of milk and eating calcium-rich dairy foods may not help women avoid bone fractures in later life and may, in fact, increase the risk. The 12-year study, which involved over 120,000 women throughout the United States, found that women who drank two or more glasses of milk per day actually had a 45 per cent higher risk of hip fractures and a 5 per cent higher risk of forearm fractures than women who drank less.[15] The way the body absorbs and handles calcium in the body is very complex. Let's take a look at why just taking additional calcium is only part of the answer.

Less Well-Known Risk Factors in Osteoporosis

- Too much protein
- Inappropriate levels of stress
- Poor intake of specific nutrients
- Poor absorption and use of specific nutrients

- Too little stomach acid
- High use of stimulants
- High intake of phytates

Too Much Protein

One of the most significant, yet less well-known risk factors for osteoporosis, according to a World Health Organization research survey, is excessive protein consumption.[16] This is for two main reasons. Protein is digested in the presence of high levels of acid (hydrochloric acid, or HCl) in the stomach; and women, particularly those over 50 years of age, often produce insufficient levels of this. HCl is also vital for releasing minerals from food, so low levels can lead to poor absorption of minerals, including calcium, magnesium and zinc, all of which are vital for bone health.

The second problem is that foods which are high in protein create strong acids in the body which has to work very hard to neutralize them. It does this by calling on its reserves of what are known as alkalizing minerals, most significantly calcium. To maintain life, the blood has to be kept very slightly alkaline, and the body will do this at all costs, even if it means calling on calcium in the bones.

Eskimos – who suffer the highest rates of osteoporosis – have a classic high-protein diet: plenty of seal meat and fish, with very few fruits and vegetables. Fruits and vegetables contain acids, but they are weak and very easy for the body to dispose of. Red meat, chicken, fish, eggs and dairy produce are all high-protein foods. The trend towards eating low-fat dairy foods may be protective to your blood vessels, but not as kind to your bones. As soon as the fat content of a food is lowered, the percentage of protein increases. So high intakes of cottage cheese and low-fat yoghurt may not be such a good idea after all. Indeed, it is not vital for humans to eat animal produce at all, though small quantities of a high quality are unlikely to do any harm. Vegans – who do not eat any animal produce – are amongst the healthiest people.

Poor Absorption

Many factors can contribute to poor absorption of minerals, besides too little stomach acid. The small intestine is lined with thousands of minute structures called villi, that waft about, maximizing the body's ability to absorb nutrients. Foods rich in gluten – wheat, rye, oats and barley – can blunt the villi, decreasing the surface area available for absorption. High intakes of dairy produce can also aggravate the gut wall, leading to poor absorption. People in cultures that do not consume dairy foods have little incidence of osteoporosis. Another major factor known to interfere with good absorption is an overgrowth in the gut of the yeast organism candida albicans that is responsible for causing thrush (see Chapter 17). Diets rich in phytates, found in wheat and soya products, can bind to important minerals in the gut like calcium, magnesium and zinc, impairing their absorption.

Too Much Stress

Just like too much protein, too much stress makes the body leach calcium from the bones. Stressors include caffeine, nicotine and physical or emotional pressure. Every time your body is stressed, a red alert signal goes out in your body. Whenever this happens calcium is called out of your bones into your blood to help prepare the body for the perceived danger. A stressful job, relationships, and/or relying on tea, coffee, chocolate and cigarettes to see you through the day will almost certainly rob your bones of calcium. To add insult to injury, the calcium is not adequately called back into the bones, as the body hardly gets a chance over the day to perceive that the emergency is truly over. As it can't keep the calcium in the blood, the body disposes of it on artery walls, in joint tissue or as part of a painful gall or kidney stone.

Sub-optimum Nutrition

For most people, sub-optimum nutrition is the rule not the exception. It can occur simply through not eating enough food; but in the modern world it is more likely to be caused by eating foods that are high in calories but not nutrients – predominantly refined foods, alcohol and confectionery. A limited diet that repetitively uses the same foods is likely to be one that is unbalanced and unable to provide all the nutrients needed for health, including bone health. It is sometimes an excess of a particular nutrient that causes the problem, in combination with low levels of other nutrients.

Calcium in Balance

Calcium needs a balance of phosphorus and magnesium to build bone effectively. Typical "junk food" diets are rich in phosphorus, which disrupts this. Dairy produce is rich in calcium, but low in magnesium. Magnesium is needed to absorb and use calcium properly in the body. Nuts, seeds and green leafy vegetables are rich sources of both. Vitamin D, the sunshine vitamin, is vital for the absorption of calcium and phosphorous and helps stop them being lost in the urine. Good weight-bearing exercise, such as walking briskly on a regular basis, is a fine way to help keep calcium in the bones.

Other Important Bone Nutrients

Nutrient	Best Food Sources
zinc	nuts, seeds and wholegrains
manganese/boron	unprocessed foods
silicon/copper	unprocessed foods
vitamin A	yellow and deep green vegetables
vitamin C	berries, potatoes, most fruit and vegetables
vitamin K	cauliflower and green vegetables
vitamin B6	fruits, vegetables, wholegrains

Osteoporosis Prevention and Reversal Plan

Prevention is far better than looking for a cure and, according to the work of Dr Lee, osteoporosis is a reversible disorder. It appears that, even for someone in their seventies, the condition can be reversed. The human body responds marvellously to being provided with the right raw materials needed for health. Here's what to do:

- Take regular exercise.
- Eat plenty of wholefoods.
- Eat plenty of nuts, seeds and yellow and green vegetables.
- Eat a varied diet that includes some soya milk, tofu and wild yam.
- Reduce animal protein to the minimum.
- Avoid "junk foods" and stimulants.
- Limit alcohol.
- Seek advice from a professional nutrition consultant to check out complicating factors like candidiasis, digestive function and individual supplement requirements.

Tests for Osteoporosis Risk

To assess your risk of osteoporosis, your GP can recommend a bone mineral density scan or a nutritionist can recommend a simple urine test.

Bone Mineral Density (BMD) Scans

Two very good techniques are available that give reliable and accurate readings. BMD scans can be requested through your medical practitioner or paid for privately. Dual photon absorptiometry (DPA) is 96–98 per cent accurate for the hips and spinal column. Dual energy X-ray absorptiometry (DEXA) is also 96–98 per cent accurate but does use low-dose X-rays. These detect osteoporosis at moderately advanced stages.

Pyrilinks-D

This is a urine test that measures deoxypyridinoline (Dpd), a crosslink of collagen found in bone. This test enables your medical practitioner or nutritionist to identify and monitor your risk of bone loss. Dpd is a specific marker for bone resorption, i.e. how quickly old bone is cleared. The test is non-invasive and convenient and can demonstrate response to therapy as early as one month in. Pyrilinks-D is said to identify bone loss early in menopause. Results of a 22-month study involving elderly and pre-menopausal women with elevated Pyrilinks-D values showed double the risk of hip fracture.[17] Pyrilinks-D values combined with BMD scans predict risk even more accurately.

It is important to remember that osteoporosis is a complex condition – it is very much a case of detective work to identify the underlying factors in each individual. For best results we recommend that you work with a nutrition consultant and your medical practitioner.

CHAPTER 13

···

HOW TO PREVENT BREAST DISEASE

Of all cancers, that of the breast is the most prevalent and the most common cause of death in women; throughout the world, it is the third most common cancer and it is on the increase. One in eleven women in the UK and one in eight in the USA develop breast cancer. Each year over 30,000 women in Britain are diagnosed as having the disease and over 15,000 die of it. That is 300 deaths a week.

The fear of developing breast cancer is a reality for many women, particularly if they have a family history of the condition. A lot of these women are aware that the chance of developing breast cancer is more than slim but are unclear about what factors are involved and how to minimize the risk.

WHAT ARE THE CONTRIBUTORY FACTORS?

With so many changes in our diet, environment and lifestyle this century, it is difficult to pinpoint the factors that contribute to breast cancer. Women who have children later in life are associated with a higher risk, as are women who do not have children at all, possibly because of the lack of extra progesterone that is present during pregnancy. More recently, smoking has been linked to the development of breast cancer. Other factors that have been shown to correlate with an increased risk include rapid growth and greater adult height, high body mass, adult weight gain, alcohol, total fat, meat, animal protein intake, and consumption of DDT residues. Increasing intake of fruits, vegetables, fiber and carotenoids is considered to be protective, as is physical activity. Less conclusive, though data is accumulating, is the evidence for the protective role of vitamin C, isoflavones and complex carbohydrates (see Part 5).

Synthetic Hormones

Synthetic hormones are strongly linked to the development of breast cancer: there is a 50 per cent greater risk in women who took the Pill before the age of 20. The *New England Medical Journal* reported that, "Studies over a six-year period have shown that the longer HRT is taken there is a fourfold increased risk for developing breast cancer." Progestogens (synthetic progesterone) also assist the development of blood vessels which may encourage the spread of cancer.

High Estrogen Levels

About 80 per cent of breast cancers are termed "estrogen receptor positive." Breast cancer tends to be most prevalent when estrogen dominance is likely, i.e. during the five to ten years before menopause. It is more likely to occur when estrogen levels are high and progesterone levels low. When women under 40 have their ovaries removed (the ovaries being the primary site for the production of estrogen in pre-menopausal women) the incidence of breast cancer is significantly reduced.[18] Men treated with estrogens for cancer of the prostate also show an increased incidence of breast cancer.[19] Xenoestrogens are increasingly being recognized as a likely link in the growing incidence of breast cancer.

The Fat Factor

Several studies have confirmed the link between too much dietary fat and breast cancer. It is a complex cycle, in that high body mass is associated with an increased risk; large numbers of fat cells produce more estrogen which in turn increases the person's susceptibility to accumulating more fat. Fatty tissue is also an ideal storage site for toxins such as pesticides and organochlorines. The pesticide Lindane – which has been banned in most countries, but not the UK – has been linked with an increased risk of breast cancer in agricultural areas where it is used. Cows' milk and butter are the main sources of Lindane: the cow eats grass, which has been contaminated by Lindane, and stores it in its fatty tissue, which we then consume in milk and butter.

WHAT ARE THE TREATMENTS?

Tamoxifen

Tamoxifen is an anti-estrogen drug that is commonly prescribed to women with breast cancer, and to healthy women at a high risk. It is a weak estrogen that competes with the natural estrogens at the cell receptor sites. Tamoxifen is said to be carcinogenic and to contribute to an early menopause, osteoporosis, endometrial and liver cancer and clotting diseases. In fact, the World Health Organization officially listed tamoxifen as a human carcinogen in 1996.[20] Researcher Dr Ellen Grant reported a meagre 0.7 per cent benefit for women taking tamoxifen preventatively.[21] Other researchers conclude that tamoxifen fails to meet the safety standards required for a primary prevention measure. Dr John Lee believes that using natural progesterone helps counteract the drug's negative side-effects without interfering with the clinical benefits.

Natural Progesterone

Estrogen stimulates the proliferation and division of breast cells (the greater the rate of growth, the greater the risk for cancer); while progesterone inhibits proliferation of cells in favor of the cells maturing. In January 1996 an 18-year retrospective study at Guy's Hospital, London, was reported in the *British Journal of Cancer* as showing that a raised level of progesterone at the time of tumor removal was associated with an improvement in outcome for women with operable breast cancer.[22]

Dr John Lee believes that natural progesterone is a viable treatment in the management of cancer, as it helps moderate the proliferative effect of estrogen on breast cells. He says that if the breast cancer is shown to be receptive to progesterone it is likely to respond to its balancing and anti-cancer effects.

WHICH NUTRIENTS HELP PREVENT BREAST CANCER?

Dietary Fiber

Sufficient dietary fiber – i.e. 35g daily – helps to bind used-up hormones and eliminate them, so they cannot be reactivated and reabsorbed (see Chapter 23, which discusses this more fully). Good sources of dietary fiber are wholegrains, pulses, vegetables and fruit. Animal produce contains none.

B Vitamins

B vitamins are involved in breaking down estrogen and clearing it from the liver. Ensuring your diet is rich in B vitamins, as described in the Diet for the Good Life (see Chapter 23), is critical to hormonal balance.

Antioxidant Nutrients

The activity of free oxidizing radicals, which damage cells, is a central factor in the development of cancer. Fat oxidizes in breast (and other) tissue, increasing susceptibility to cancer, so it is advisable to take the full range of antioxidant nutrients. These include vitamins A, C and E, and the minerals zinc, selenium, iron and manganese (see the chart in Chapter 25 for dosage levels).

FIBROCYSTIC BREAST DISEASE

Cysts, or lumps, in the breast occur in 20–50 per cent of women. Symptoms are tender breasts and movable cysts which are usually near the surface. The problem usually progresses until the menopause and then subsides. It is associated with too much estrogen, particularly estrone and estradiol which are extremely active stimulants of breast tissue.

Food and drinks containing the chemical methylxanthine (found in tea, coffee, cola and chocolate) have been shown in several studies to aggravate the problem. Although most cysts are benign, they indicate an increased chance of developing breast cancer. Vitamin A has been shown to help reduce breast pain and one study reduced breast cysts masses by at least 50 per cent in five patients out of ten. Several studies supplementing vitamin E up to 600iu have shown objective and subjective remissions.[23] Evening primrose oil (1500mg twice a day) has also been shown to reduce breast pain, tenderness and cyst size. Ginseng – probably because it contains small amounts of estrone, estradiol and estriol – has in some studies been linked to breast pain and tenderness. A low-salt diet helps reduce breast tenderness and swelling. Dr John Lee has found that supplementing natural progesterone, 600iu of vitamin E, 300mg of magnesium and 50mg of B6 a day has always given positive results. Follow the Diet for the Good Life as described in Chapter 23.

CHAPTER 14

HOW TO PREVENT UTERINE AND CERVICAL DISEASE

Many of the serious health problems that relate to the female reproductive tract have been steadily increasing, though recent reports indicate that cancers of the uterus, ovaries and cervix are showing a decline in developed countries.[24] Cervical cancer is the second most common cancer in women, while endometrial (the lining of the uterus) is the eighth most common, and ovarian is the seventh most common. Taken together, these three cancers result in over 8 per cent of all new cases of cancer in a year. Any decline has been attributed to widespread screening programs. Although scientific data has not proved a conclusive link with diet, researchers have noted that high intakes of vegetables and fruits possibly reduce risk; and they have found a possible association with a high intake of saturated fat in both ovarian and endometrial cancer.[25]

Less serious but extremely debilitating problems – from painful and heavy periods to endometriosis and pelvic inflammatory disease – affect women on a daily or cyclical basis. Endometriosis has been described as "the hidden epidemic." One in 10 women suffer from this condition during their reproductive years. So let's take a look at how optimizing your nutritional status can play a part in the management and prevention of these problems.

MENSTRUAL PROBLEMS

Painful Periods

Painful periods are not uncommon, particularly in young women before they have had a baby. Many women gain relief from following a general optimum nutrition program as outlined in the Diet for the Good Life (Chapter 23) and dealing with allergies and/or candidiasis (see Chapters 16 and 17).

The muscles of the uterus, like other muscles in the body, can become unbalanced in their ability to contract and relax. During a period these muscles are working extra-hard to shed the inner lining of the uterus. Calcium and magnesium are the two major nutrients needed to control this process. Eating healthy foods rich in calcium and magnesium, and taking supplements, has helped many women. Essential polyunsaturated oils, vitamin E and the mineral zinc may also help. It is worth taking supplements to boost your intake of these nutrients. Essential polyunsaturated oils are particularly likely to help if the pain is associated with a heavy blood loss that has a tendency to clot. These oils make a type of prostaglandin that controls blood thickness. Vitamin E can also help reduce cramps. Cutting down on red meat and dairy produce should help too, as these high-fat foods can interfere with prostaglandin balance.

The contraceptive pill is often recommended for period pains. However, nutritionally oriented doctors do not recommend this approach, as the Pill interferes with the working of many essential nutrients. Many women recover from painful periods naturally, with help from the same nutrients that are depleted by the Pill.

The muscles of the uterus, like other muscles in the body, can become unbalanced in their ability to contract and relax. During a period these muscles are working extra-hard to shed the inner lining of the uterus. Calcium and magnesium are the two major nutrients needed to control this process. Calcium helps the muscle to contract and magnesium helps the muscle to relax. Many diets that rely heavily on dairy produce are rich in calcium but relatively poor in magnesium. Including nuts, seeds and dark green leafy vegetables into your diet often helps as these foods are rich in both calcium and magnesium.

Heavy Periods

Follow the Diet for the Good Life (Chapter 23) and, with the help of a nutrition consultant, test for any food intolerances. Some women find that their periods get heavier in the first few months of an anti-candida diet (see Chapter 17), but it usually settles down.

One study showed that heavy periods may be caused by a deficiency of vitamin A.[26] Vitamin A levels appear to fluctuate over the month, indicating a correlation with fluctuating female hormones. Another study clearly indicated that women with heavy periods had less than half the normal levels of vitamin A in their bloodstream. Researchers found that, when treating heavy periods with high levels of vitamin A daily for 35 days, over half the participants' heavy periods were completely cured, and 14 more women showed a marked improvement. In all, 93 per cent improved. Sometimes it may not be that vitamin A is actually deficient. Vitamin A is a fat-soluble vitamin which is stored in the liver; zinc and vitamin E are needed to make use of reserves, so a lack of these nutrients can lead to apparent vitamin A deficiency.

The contraceptive pill often creates a high level of vitamin A in the blood, and, while taking the Pill, a woman's periods are usually fine. The Pill creates this high level of vitamin A in the blood by moving it from its store in the liver. However, when a woman stops taking the Pill, the level of vitamin A in the blood can fall dramatically, consequently depleting stores in the liver. It is therefore common to experience heavy periods after stopping the Pill.

Vitamin C and bioflavonoids have been shown to help control heavy periods. Bioflavonoids are found mainly just beneath the surface skin of fruit. It is unclear whether low iron levels are an effect, as well as a cause, of heavy periods, but correcting them is an essential part of any program. Taking vitamin C with iron-rich foods increases the absorption of iron.

Irregular Periods

Depending on the cause, irregular periods can be perfectly normal. Towards the menopause, it is to be expected that periods will become irregular; and they stop altogether during pregnancy. If your periods are either absent or irregular, and you do not come into either of these categories, it is worth checking out the cause. Absent or irregular periods are associated with low weight, strenuous exercise, anorexia nervosa, taking the contraceptive pill, or extreme stress. Extreme stress can lead to either missed periods or more frequent periods. Follow the Diet for the Good Life (see Chapter 23).

OTHER DISORDERS AFFECTING THE REPRODUCTIVE SYSTEM

Fibroids

Fibroids are the most common growths in the female reproductive system. They are benign, firm, round lumps (usually more than one) that attach themselves to the muscular wall of the uterus. They often grow to the size of a grapefruit and routinely disappear after the menopause. They are, however, one of the most common reasons why pre-menopausal women have their uteri removed. Symptoms are irregular, heavy and painful periods, while the weight of the fibroids can weaken the pelvic floor muscles, leading to stress incontinence. The usual treatment is to remove them surgically.

Fibroids are a result of estrogen dominance, so when levels fall at the menopause the fibroids shrink. According to Dr John Lee, when the estrogen dominance is addressed by using natural progesterone, the fibroid tumors normally decrease in size and can usually be kept at a minimum until the menopause when they will naturally shrivel up. Estrogen dominance can be easily detected by a simple saliva test to measure estrogen and progesterone levels. Follow the recommendations for fibrocystic breasts on page 93.

Ovarian Cysts

Ovarian cysts result from an egg failing to develop and be released normally. They can grow to the size of a golf ball and create considerable pain but sometimes produce no symptoms at all. After ovulation fails, the developing egg continues to grow, under the influence of follicle stimulating hormone (FSH). Each month, the rise of FSH is followed by a surge of luteinizing hormone (LH), which causes the site of the follicle to swell, stretching the surface of the ovary, causing pain and possibly bleeding at the site. Treatment may involve surgery.

It has been suggested that when zinc is in short supply certain types of cysts can develop, possibly because zinc is required for the growth of the egg. The use of infertility drugs has also been implicated because some of these drugs block estrogen receptors and increase the output of FSH and LH even though women are failing to ovulate.

Dr John Lee has found that supplementing natural progesterone from day 10 to day 26 of the cycle for a few months is
often enough to shrink the cysts and no further treatment is
required. Taking progesterone from day 10 effectively suppresses ovulation and gives the ovaries time to rest and repair.
Follow the Diet for the Good Life (see Chapter 23).

Endometriosis

Endometriosis is a very common and painful disease which is
thought to affect one in 10 women. Its cause remains
unknown. Small fragments of endometrial tissue (uterine lining) migrate into the muscular wall of the uterus and out
through the fallopian tubes. The fragments can be found on
the surface of the ovaries and in the pelvic organs, including
the bowel. Endometrial tissue has been found in many distant
sites of the body, well away from the uterus.

In response to the natural fluctuations of estrogens and
progesterone, the fragments swell up with blood during the
month and also bleed at the time of menstruation and at other
times during the cycle. This can cause considerable pain,
which often starts shortly before menstruation and does not
subside until it is finished. Some women find that their pain
increases at the time of ovulation. Sexual intercourse and
emptying the bowel are also commonly painful. Endometriosis is a frequent cause of infertility and heavy and
irregular bleeding. About 50 per cent of women investigated
for infertility are found to have endometriosis. One study
showed that women who had taken the Pill had nearly twice
the incidence of endometriosis as women who had never
taken it.[27] Pregnancy often retards the progress of the disease
and sometimes cures it. The condition is usually treated by
synthetic progestogens to simulate a pregnant state.

Inflammation occurs around the sites of the endometrial
deposits and research using fish oils has been shown to shrink

the size of the deposits. Animal fats produce a substance in the body that promotes inflammation and should be reduced in the diet. Vitamin C also helps to reduce inflammation. As well as having anti-inflammatory properties, vitamin E has been shown in trials to reduce pain in the lower part of the back. Vitamin B6, biotin and B3 have been seen to have anti-inflammatory effects which simultaneously help to reduce pain.

Magnesium acts to relax muscles and can be helpful in reducing the very painful cramps at the time of the period (see also the nutrients recommended for painful periods on page 96). DL Phenylalanine (DLPA) is an amino acid that has been reported to help relieve pain in 60 per cent of those that try it.[28] DLPA is available on prescription.

Reducing exposure to xenoestrogens is advisable too, as estrogen dominance is also linked to endometriosis. Recent research by the American Endometriosis Association has associated the pesticide dioxin with the epidemic of endometriosis. Pesticides interfere with the action of choline, a B vitamin that helps the liver break down estrogen. Food is the largest source of dioxin, animal fat being a major contributor. The USA minimum risk is set at 0.0064 units a day, whereas the UK authorities accept a dioxin intake of 10 units a day. Dioxins are also associated with an increased risk of cancer.

Dr John Lee has had considerable success in treating endometriosis with natural progesterone which helps to stop further proliferation of the endometrial cells created by estrogen. He recommends that natural progesterone cream is used from day 6 to day 26 of the cycle. Over four to six months, the pains usually gradually subside (though they do not always disappear entirely); as the monthly bleeding becomes less, so the inflamed sites can heal. Endometriosis usually subsides at the menopause.

Pelvic Inflammatory Disease (PID)

PID is a serious inflammation of the uterus and fallopian tubes which can give rise to pelvic abscesses, pain and infertility. It is usually treated with antibiotics and surgery is not uncommon. Infection first occurs in the vagina and cervix and can ascend into the endometrium in the uterus and along the fallopian tubes.

Prevention is better than cure. Increasing the body's resistance to opportunistic infections like candida and chlamydia is a high priority. This involves boosting your immune system and dealing with stress. Vital nutrients are vitamins C, E, A, B6, and calcium, magnesium, zinc, selenium and essential oils. Follow the Diet For the Good Life (see Chapter 23).

As a woman nears the menopause, her estrogen levels decline, increasing her susceptibility to vaginal infections as her mucus production changes. Natural hormones may offer some protection, although women on the Pill are more susceptible. Beta-carotene and vitamins C and E are needed for normal mucus production.

Cervical Erosions and/or Dysplasia (Abnormal Cervical Cells)

Hormone imbalance and folic acid deficiency have been linked to both of these problems. A study showed success in 100 per cent of cases following treatment with 10mg of folic acid daily.[29] Another study involved 47 women with mild or moderate dysplasia, who had been taking the combined pill for at least six months, receiving either 10mg of folate daily or a placebo. After three months, cervical biopsies showed significant improvement only in those women receiving folate. In seven women the dysplasia disappeared. Four of the women receiving the placebo showed progression to cancer.

Low levels of vitamin A, vitamin C and the mineral selenium have been associated with cervical dysplasia. Women consuming less than average vitamin A and beta-carotene were three times as likely to develop severe dysplasia and three to four times more likely to develop cancer. According to Dr John Lee, when folic acid is given in doses of 3–5mg, alongside 50mg of vitamin B6 and 300mg of magnesium, recovery usually takes place in one to two cycles. If recovery is delayed then using progesterone or estriol intravaginally during the month between periods should help restore normal cervical tissue.

The cells of the cervix are extremely hormone-sensitive. Levels of progestogen low enough not to alter the cells of the lining of the uterus, have been shown to change the cells lining the cervix. Progestogens dry up cervical secretions, and this may be part of the reason why cancer of the cervix develops quickly in the presence of cervical infections. Smoking is highly correlated with cervical cancer.

Endometrial Cancer

The first life-threatening health problem associated with taking estrogen-only HRT was the increased risk of developing endometrial cancer. It is now also known that, if a woman who has not had a hysterectomy is given only estrogen, it increases her chance of developing endometrial cancer up to 20 times – a risk that increases the longer she takes HRT. Estrogens cause rapid growth of endometrial cells, which could encourage cancer growth. To limit this danger, it was recommended that a progestogen be taken with the estrogen, and tests showed that this combined hormone therapy could prevent endometrial cancer. One side-effect of taking progestogen, however, is withdrawal bleeding, which is treated by giving continuous progestogen, which in turn can lead to breakthrough bleeding, ultimately negating its protective effects against endometrial cancer.

The conclusion was that women who have not had a hysterectomy should always receive estrogens alongside progesterone or a progestogen to prevent endometrial cancer. The risk factors for developing endometrial cancer correlate well with those of estrogen dominance. Endometrial cancer only tends to occur during the 5 to 10 years before menopause when anovulatory cycles are common. Taking dietary phytoestrogens (explained in Chapter 24) and natural progesterone during these years before menopause can significantly reduce the incidence of endometrial cancer, according to Dr John Lee.

There is now clear evidence that an excess of calories – particularly in fats – increases estrogen levels and this helps to explain why there is a higher incidence of these cancers in the West, due to our high-fat diet.

Ovarian Cancer

The incidence of ovarian cancer, which is thought to afflict 2 per cent of women, increases with age, and is most prevalent amongst educated, higher social class, white women. Research at the John Hopkins University School, USA, involving 240,073 women, indicates that the long-term use of estrogen replacement therapy (in HRT) may increase the risk of fatal ovarian cancer.[30] Dr Ellison of Harvard University suggests that the abnormal levels of estrogen may be linked to the current epidemic of breast and ovarian cancer. He also goes on to propose that the high hormone levels are a reflection of over-eating and under-exercising. Follow the Diet for the Good Life as described in Chapter 23.

CHAPTER 15

BEATING THE SUGAR BLUES

Most of us like sweet foods – in nature they are usually safe – and modern food processing has cashed in on our inclination towards sweet foods. From early infancy, when sugar is added to baby drinks and foods we become hooked on the desire for something sweet.

In the 1820s the average daily intake of sugar amounted to two teaspoons, which is the amount of glucose (sugar) that we have in our blood at any one time. By the 1980s the average intake of sugar had risen to an amazing 38 teaspoons a day! When you consider that a Mars Bar contains around 15 teaspoons of sugar, and a cola drink around 7 teaspoons, and then what is added to tea, coffee, cereals, biscuits and cakes, it soon adds up.

However, we do not need to eat sugar to increase the level of glucose in our blood. Stress, in all its guises, does this very efficiently, without us ever having to put a teaspoon of sugar into our mouths. A difficult day at work or at home with the children, having a cup of coffee and a cigarette, eating too much red meat or salt, taking in foods that we react to allergically, or just watching a horror movie all effectively raise our blood sugar level.

THE STRESS CONNECTION

In modern times, it is difficult not to be stressed. Just living shoulder to shoulder in suburbia and commuting to town every day is stressful. We all experience stress differently: some of us enjoy stress; others perform badly under it; and there are some people who feel stressed because there isn't enough stress in their lives.

Whatever the stressor, the body will respond to it in the same way: by releasing a variety of chemicals to deal with the situation. The adrenal glands release adrenalin, which releases the stores of sugar into the blood and cortisol (which is needed to help regulate glucose and energy balance as well as moderate any inflammatory reactions). The released sugar is taken from the blood to the cells, to be burnt for energy to deal with a perceived emergency. A substance called glucose tolerance factor (GTF) helps the hormone insulin take the sugar into the cells.

As part of this reaction, calcium is released from its store in the bones in preparation for an immediate "fight" by increasing the heart rate and the ability of the muscles to contract. Calcium is also involved in blood clotting which would be necessary in the event of any injury in the "fight."

The problem is that we are not in a real "fight." More often than not, we are just dealing with another work or family pressure or another cup of coffee. If we were dealing with a true emergency, like stopping a young child from running across the road at the wrong time, then the chemicals released to deal with the situation would be appropriate and the body would use them up. After the emergency was over, the chemistry would settle down and the body would regain its balance.

Modern-day stressors are continually present in our lives. Almost every hour of every day, we are likely to be stressing our bodies for one reason or another. So, regaining our chemical balance is difficult because our bodies do not receive a clear message that the emergency is over.

It is important to consider the body as inherently wise, but its wisdom is moment by moment, not long-term. It acts according to the immediate priorities. So how do our bodies react to these "fake emergencies":

- If the sugar that is released is not used for energy it can be converted to fat which may end up on artery walls, be converted to cholesterol (which may also stick to artery walls), or it may be stored as body fat.

- If the calcium that is released is not properly instructed to return to the bones after the perceived emergency then it, too, may end up on artery walls (contributing to hardening of the arteries), or be deposited into joint tissue (contributing to arthritis).

- If the calcium is not returned to the bones efficiently then the risk of osteoporosis is increased.

The body has to respond in this way. It has no other option, because excess sugar in the blood would be life-threatening. Similarly, the level of calcium circulating in the blood has to be kept within strict limits to maintain life. The body is effectively dumping dangerous material from circulation into places where it can do no immediate harm. The fact that coronary artery disease, obesity, arthritis or osteoporosis may develop years hence, is not relevant at the time.

THE SYMPTOMS OF GLUCOSE IMBALANCE

The problems are not all long-term ones. Many people experience unpleasant symptoms on a daily basis for years as a result of adrenal stress. When the body responds to an adrenal stimulant with a surge of sugar entering the bloodstream it makes us feel good. But what usually happens half an hour or so later is that we experience the downside. Too much insulin is released to bring the blood sugar level down. The symptoms, such as irritability, anxiety, depression, mood swings and poor concentration, mainly affect our mental well-being.

When we are not physically active, the majority of sugar in the body feeds the brain, so mental well-being is affected first when our blood sugar levels drop. Having relied on artificial stimulation throughout the day, it is not uncommon to find it difficult to sleep at night. The body may be tired, but the mind is still racing. Equally, it can be difficult to get going in the morning until we have had our first "fix" of tea or coffee or a cigarette.

Symptoms of glucose imbalance are irritability, anxiety, insomnia, depression, dizziness, mood swings, poor concentration, food cravings, irritability after six hours without food, excessive thirst, addiction to sweet food, cold hands, need for excessive sleep during the day, drowsiness during the day, lack of energy, need for more than eight hours sleep at night, rarely awake within 20 minutes of rising, need for something to get going in the morning like tea, coffee or cigarette, excessive sweating, avoidance of exercise due to tiredness.

As most of us do not like feeling this way, the tendency is to turn to another cup of coffee or tea, a chocolate bar or cigarette to pick us up again. This vicious cycle can keep us addicted all our lives unless we know better or choose to do something about it.

THE HORMONE FACTOR

Adrenal stress is inextricably tied up with sex hormone imbalance. As described in Part 1, the stress hormone cortisol competes with the same receptor sites as progesterone, so the net effect of being permanently stressed is less active progesterone. Since cortisol can also increase the production of estrogen, prolonged stress can contribute to estrogen dominance. Estrogen also encourages the body to lay down fat. In addition, high cortisol levels can reduce the production of an immunoglobulin called secretory IgA that protects the membranes of the gut, the airways and the urinary tract, and increase the risk of having a leaky gut as described on page 39. So it is clear that stress can wreak havoc in the body and can be a significant contributory factor in the development of degenerative diseases.

Given that most of our lives are stressful to varying degrees, it is essential that this factor is addressed as part of any program to manage sex hormone imbalances.

Breaking the sugar habit

This is easier said than done, as addressing this problem goes to the heart of modern lifestyles and addictions. However, if you can break the habit, the benefits to your health and quality of life will far outweigh the supposed pleasure of the addictions. Like most other things in life, it is a matter of choice.

The Diet – Step 1

The easiest place to start is to pay attention to your general diet. The essential first steps are regular meals (i.e. five a day – three main and two snacks), and eating nutritious wholefoods that release their natural sugar content slowly and good quality protein. Having protein with each intake of food helps the body to handle sugar more efficiently, as it stimulates the production of the hormone glucagon that helps to keep blood sugar levels under control and also helps the body burn fat for energy. Good quality types of protein to include in the three main meals of the day are: free-range meat, free-range eggs, organic dairy produce, a little fish, tofu and pulses. Nuts and seeds are good as snacks. Ensure that you eat plenty of vegetables with each intake, as they help to keep the body in its natural alkaline state.

Although fruit is good, an excess can aggravate blood sugar problems. Bananas, dates and grapes release their sugar content rapidly, while a crunchy apple or pear are much more slow-releasing. Two crisp apples or pears a day should be fine. Avoid tinned, dried and overly ripe fruit. Dilute fruit juices with an equal quantity of water. Wherever possible, replace wheat with rye, oats or a high-protein grain called quinoa (which cooks like rice).

The Diet – Step 2

Foods that you may be reacting to allergically can upset your blood sugar levels. As described in Chapter 16, the common offenders are wheat, dairy produce, citrus fruits and yeast. If you think this applies to you then follow the guidelines in that chapter. Be sure that you replace the offending foods with suitable alternatives.

The Diet – Step 3

Now comes the crunch. Time to give up the caffeine. Whether you are drinking two or 20 cups of tea and coffee a day, and eating one or seven bars of chocolate a week, this is the time to let go. The most effective way in our experience is to just choose a day and stop. But if you do this, expect to experience withdrawal symptoms for a few days. Taking the supplements described below should help to modify the effects of withdrawal symptoms like headaches, irritability and muscle aches. Ensuring that you keep to Steps 1 and 2 while withdrawing from caffeine should also make it easier. If you are a smoker, then it is much more likely that you will successfully quit this habit, having improved your diet, made it more alkaline and dealt with any other addictions.

Nutritional Supplements

We recommend that the following supplements are taken from day one of starting a program to address the sugar blues. In our experience, clients do much better when supported with extra nutrients that are known to assist in blood sugar control.

Vitamins B1, B2, B3, B5, vitamin C, and the minerals magnesium, manganese, iron and copper, are needed to turn glucose (sugar) into energy. Vitamin B6 and the mineral zinc are required for the production of adrenalin. Vitamin B3 and the mineral chromium are part of GTF which helps the action of insulin. Vitamin B5 and vitamin C are needed to support the adrenal glands. A balance of calcium and magnesium is required so that each can be used effectively.

Supplementing a high-strength multivitamin and mineral that gives 50mg of the B vitamins would be a good way to start. In addition, 1g of vitamin C, 100mcg of chromium, and 600mg of calcium, with a balance of 400mg of magnesium, would be a supportive program.

CHAPTER 16

THE ALLERGY CONNECTION

The classic definition of an allergy is "any idiosyncratic reaction where the immune system is clearly involved." Classical allergies – commonly to foods like shellfish and peanuts – are quite easily identified. They often present as asthma, eczema, hayfever and hives and may even be life-threatening by causing immediate reactions like swelling in the throat. They are recognized by a marker in the blood which is an antibody called immunoglobulin E (IgE).

Nutrition consultants have for many years helped certain clients improve their health by recommending that they avoid regular foods in the diet like wheat, dairy, citrus fruits, yeast and caffeine, even though there is no evidence of a classical allergy. Results have borne out the value of recommending such avoidance. However, the emerging view now is that most allergies are not IgE-based. There is a new school of thought and a new generation of allergy tests has been designed to detect allergies. These involve another marker known as immunoglobulin G (IgG).

According to Dr James Braly, a director of Immuno Laboratories, which developed the IgG ELISA test (an allergy test that determines to which foods a person produces abnormal amounts of IgG):

Food allergy is not rare, nor are the effects limited to the air passages, the skin and digestive tract. Most food allergies are delayed reactions, taking anywhere from an hour to three days to show themselves, and are therefore much harder to detect. Delayed food allergy appears to be simply the inability of your digestive tract to prevent large quantities of partially digested and undigested food from entering the bloodstream.

Many food allergies are likely to occur when the lining of the gut wall is leakier than it should be (see page 39). Foods can act as a local irritant to the gut wall and make it more porous. If larger particles of food escape into the bloodstream through the gut wall, the immune system sees them as foreign and sets up an inflammatory reaction. Headaches, joint pains, flatulence, bloating, mood swings, water retention and food cravings may result. Food allergens may also give the body a stress signal, setting up an inappropriate physical response.

It is now well established that many, if not the majority, of food intolerances do not produce immediate symptoms, but have a delayed, cumulative effect, often two or three days after the food has been eaten. This, of course, makes them hard to detect by observation. Because they do not present in a classical way, in the form of asthma or hives, for example, many people do not realize that their unpleasant symptoms could be associated with a food that they are eating regularly. IgG reactions are associated with overuse of particular foods in the diet.

WHEAT AND DAIRY PRODUCTS

The two most common allergens in the U. S. are wheat and dairy products. As a result of busy lifestyles and dependence on convenience foods, many people are completely unaware of the origins of their food.

Wheat is the cheapest and easiest grain to grow, and its

flour is not only used to bake bread, cakes, biscuits, etc but also as a filler in many processed foods. The quantity of wheat in the average person's diet is therefore much higher than it was 50 years ago, particularly as so many of us are partial to a quick pasta or pizza dish in front of the TV after a hard day's work.

It is quite common now, not only because of convenience foods, but also as part of an increasing emphasis on healthy eating (even for vegetarians), to be very dependent on wheat and dairy produce. For example, it is not untypical to have bran flakes and skimmed milk for breakfast, a wholemeal low-fat cheese sandwich for lunch, and a wholemeal pizza or pasta dish for supper, interspersed with fruits and vegetables. Effectively, the main food components are wheat and dairy for breakfast, lunch and supper, just assembled in different forms.

Strangely, it is quite usual for people to crave a food that they are reacting to. If it is a slice of bread or a biscuit that you crave, then consider that you may be reacting to wheat. Similarly, if it is a glass of milk or a lump of cheese that gets you raiding the fridge, consider a dairy allergy. Common symptoms are mood swings, irritability, foggy brain, flatulence, bloating, water retention and joint pains.

TESTING FOR ALLERGIES

If you suspect that you are reacting to a food, try avoiding all wheat and dairy produce for two weeks. After a few days of withdrawal symptoms, which may include headaches, muscle aches and mood swings, you should start to feel better. After two weeks, eat a large amount of wheat at one meal and observe how you feel over the next three days. Five minutes before you eat the food, take your pulse, having been at rest for at least 15 minutes. Take your pulse again, five minutes, 15 minutes, 30 minutes and one hour after eating the wheat.

If your pulse increases by 10 over that period, that is an indication that you have reacted to the food. Three days later, follow the same procedure to test for dairy produce. If you find your symptoms get worse, avoid the food for a further three months and then try again. If there is no reaction, bring small amounts slowly back into your diet. Any food that you suspect may be a problem can be tested in this way.

It is very important that you replace these major foods with suitable alternatives that will replace the nutrients lost by their exclusion. Read labels on food to ensure that they are free from wheat and dairy produce. Alternatives to wheat include corn pasta, rye pasta, rice pasta, rice cakes, rye bread, rye crackers, oat cakes, brown rice, wholegrain cornflakes, porridge oats and millet flakes. Alternatives to dairy produce include soya milk, rice milk, oat milk, tofu, soya cheese, nuts, seeds and green leafy vegetables. If you tell the assistant in a healthfood shop that you are avoiding wheat and dairy produce then they will be able to show you some alternatives.

It is possible to react to any food. A nutrition consultant will be able to recommend a full allergy screen for you, if you believe allergies are part of your health problem, and the simple method described above proves inconclusive.

CHAPTER 17

CONQUERING CANDIDA

Candidiasis is the excessive growth of a yeast organism called Candida albicans, which is a normal inhabitant of the bowel. The large intestine is home to 1.3–1.8 kg (3–4 lb) of organisms, most of which, in the right balance, are very important to our health. However, given the right conditions, opportunistic organisms like Candida albicans can take over, leaving the sufferer feeling ill all over.

WHAT CAUSES CANDIDIASIS?

This yeast is not harmful unless it is encouraged to multiply. It flourishes on a diet of sugars, yeasts and moulds, in foods such as alcohol, confectionery, processed foods, dried fruits, bread, mushrooms, Marmite, pickles, vinegar and anything fermented.

Indiscriminate use of antibiotics reduces the number of friendly organisms in the gut, creating more room for the unfriendly ones. Hormone treatments and other steroid medications can depress the immune system, enabling the Candida organism to take a hold.

If this yeast organism is allowed to proliferate it develops a root, becoming fungal in form; and the ecological function of fungi is to recycle organic material. Erica White, author of *The Beat Candida Cookbook*, writes that, for Candida, "The human body is a pile of organic material and, given half the chance, it will take advantage of a depressed immune system or impoverished gut flora and start to recycle us."

WHAT ARE THE EFFECTS OF CANDIDIASIS?

In the fungal form the organism is able to penetrate the gut wall, making it leakier than it should be. This way, Candida and the toxins it produces enter the bloodstream, along with other unwanted substances, increasing the risk of food allergy, hormonal dysfunction, bowel problems, skin problems, muscle pain, fatigue, thrush and emotional problems. Once in the bloodstream, Candida tends to settle in weak spots, for example in the joints where it can cause pain.

Many of the symptoms of candidiasis arise as a result of an increased level of toxins in the blood and include: headaches, irritability, anxiety, depression, joint aches, insomnia, anal irritation, bloating, flatulence, mood swings, dizziness, and oral and vaginal thrush.

WHAT TREATMENTS ARE AVAILABLE?

The aim of any program to treat candidiasis is to starve the organism through dietary restriction, re-establish a healthy gut flora, heal the gut and then target the organism directly with an anti-fungal agent. Depending on the severity of the invasion, the process can be lengthy and expensive. Because of its intensity and cost, we recommend that you take one of two tests before you embark on the program to find out whether candidiasis is the problem. One is a stool test which gives a quantative evaluation of the presence of the organism in the gut. The second is an immunoglobulin test which shows up any immune reaction to Candida albicans. We believe that the second test is the most conclusive.

Apart from laboratory tests, the following questionnaire is

a good indicator of the problem. It's important to note, though, that similar symptoms can arise from other organisms in the gut which will not be completely eliminated by an anti-Candida program. There are more comprehensive stool tests that can detect some of the less common invaders of the gut. A nutrition consultant can work with you and recommend the appropriate tests to find out which particular organisms are contributing to the problem.

THE CANDIDA QUESTIONNAIRE

History

1 Have you ever taken tetracycline or other antibiotics for a month or longer?
2 Have you, at any time in your life, taken other broad-spectrum antibiotics for respiratory, urinary or other infections (for two months or longer, or in shorter courses four or more times in a one-year period)?
3 Have you, at any time in your life, been bothered by persistent prostatitis, vaginitis or other problems affecting your reproductive organs?
4 Have you taken birth control pills for more than two years?
5 Have you taken cortisone-type drugs for more than a month?
6 Does exposure to perfumes, insecticides, cigarette smoke and other chemicals provoke noticeable symptoms?
7 Are your symptoms worse on damp, muggy days or in mouldy places?
8 Do you have athlete's foot, ringworm, "jock itch" or other chronic fungal infections of the skin or nails?
9 Do you crave sugar, bread or alcoholic beverages?

Score 2 points for each "yes" answer.

Symptoms

1 Do you often experience fatigue or lethargy?
2 Do you ever have the feeling of being drained?
3 Do you suffer from depression?
4 Do you have a poor memory?
5 Do you ever experience feeling "spacey" or "unreal"?
6 Do you suffer from an inability to make decisions?
7 Do you experience numbness, burning or tingling?
8 Do you ever get headaches or migraines?
9 Do you suffer from muscle aches?
10 Do you have muscle weakness or paralysis?
11 Do you have pain and/or swelling in your joints?
12 Do you suffer from abdominal pain?
13 Do you get constipation and/or diarrhea?
14 Do you suffer from bloating, belching or intestinal gas?
15 Do you have troublesome vaginal burning, itching or discharge?
16 Do you suffer from prostatitis or impotence?
17 Do you ever experience a loss of sexual desire or feeling?
18 Do you suffer from endometriosis or infertility?
19 Do you have cramps or other menstrual irregularities?
20 Do you get premenstrual tension?
21 Do you ever have attacks of anxiety or crying?
22 Do you suffer from cold hands or feet and/or chilliness?
23 Do you get shaky or irritable when hungry?

Score 1 point for each "yes" answer.

Add up your total score.

If you score **above 30** there's a strong likelihood that you have candidiasis. If you score **above 20** there's a possibility that you have a degree of candidiasis. We recommend that you see a nutrition consultant and have the appropriate tests to find out if candidiasis is your problem.

Anti-Candida Diet

This involves avoiding sugars, yeasts and moulds (including yeasted bread), alcohol, cheese, mushrooms, Marmite, pickles, vinegar, dried fruits, over-ripe fruits, and anything fermented for three to six months, depending on the severity of the problem. Some practitioners recommend a total avoidance of fruit but in our experience this has rarely been necessary, and most of our clients tolerate two crisp green apples a day. Starving the organism considerably reduces the activity in the gut and, while awaiting test results, enables some improvement to take place. For the first month we recommend that you stick with the diet only.

Healing the Gut

If the gut is found to be leaky, it is necessary to use agents like butyric acid and glutamine which are the two major energy sources for the gut wall. Addressing the healing of the gut before actively destroying the Candida organism itself usually leads to fewer "die-off" reactions (see below).

Re-establishing a Healthy Gut Flora

This is done at the same time as healing the gut. Prebiotics, like fructo-oligosaccharides, are recommended first to stimulate the growth of friendly bacteria rather than opportunistic unwanted organisms. Prebiotics should be followed by a course of probiotics, such as Lactobacillus acidophilus. We recommend that prebiotics and probiotics are taken for six months. These are available as nutritional supplements.

Anti-fungal Therapy

Three months into the program we recommend that an anti-fungal agent, such as caprylic acid, is introduced.

Waiting three months allows the dietary restrictions to reduce the activity of the Candida, gives the gut wall time to heal and generally brings about an improvement in health. Caprylic acid targets the organism directly in a mass "slaughter," which causes the release of toxins in what is known as "die-off" reaction. At this stage the sufferer is more able to tolerate the "die-off" without feeling too sick. Although this may be slower than targeting the organism with caprylic acid from the start, it usually gives the sufferer a smoother ride.

It is worth retesting at the end of the program for the presence of Candida and the health of the gut wall. In our experience, if the program does not include nutrients to heal the gut wall, the problem is likely to recur when a more "normal" diet is resumed.

POINTS TO REMEMBER

- Thrush is not necessarily an indicator of candidiasis.

- It is very difficult to treat candidiasis successfully if taking the contraceptive pill.

- It is very difficult to treat candidiasis successfully if smoking.

- Seek expert advice if you are pregnant or considering pregnancy and think that you may have candidiasis.

- Work with a nutrition consultant wherever possible if you think you have candidiasis, as the symptoms are so diverse that they can easily be mistaken for true hormone imbalances.

PART 4

NATURAL VERSUS SYNTHETIC HORMONES

CHAPTER 18

ESTROGEN AND PROGESTERONE EXPLAINED

Throughout a woman's life there is a strong case for prescribing synthetic hormones to treat a variety of health problems – from period pains and infertility to menopause and for contraception. It is predicted that by the year 2000 three in four women will be taking HRT. This, and the use of other synthetic hormones for the management of female health problems, is the largest human experiment ever. It is only now, several decades after their inception, that we are beginning to understand how synthetic hormones can wreak havoc with our hormone balance rather than promote it.

We need to understand how the two major female sex hormones, estrogen and progesterone, work, before we can see why synthetic hormones may not be all they are claimed to be. Hormones are messengers made in one part of the body, and released into the blood to affect some distant organ. To respond to the changing needs of the body, an intricate system controls their continuous production, breakdown and disposal.

To maximize reproductive ability, the body is designed to produce a balance of the hormones estrogen and progesterone. Estrogen is made from progesterone and the two are very similar in structure. They are closely interrelated in many ways, with generally opposite effects, and each helps the other by increasing the sensitivity of target organs.

UNDERSTANDING ESTROGEN

Estrogen is primarily produced by the ovaries; however, fat cells and the adrenal glands also make some and they become the primary producers from menopause onwards. Keeping the adrenal glands healthy, and not becoming too thin, helps ease the transition to menopause. Estrogen also helps lay down fat, so that, during times of famine, pregnant women can use their stores of fat as energy reserves.

During puberty in girls, estrogen encourages the growth and development of the breasts, uterus, underarm and pubic hair, and the fat that contributes to the typical female body shape. Estrogen also stimulates the lining of the vagina and encourages the production of vaginal secretions, making sexual intercourse more comfortable and protecting and cleansing the vagina. Once menstruation has started, estrogen is responsible in the first two weeks of the cycle for the maturation of an egg. A peak in estrogen levels around day 12 of the cycle brings about ovulation by stimulating the release of luteinizing hormone (LH).

UNDERSTANDING PROGESTERONE

Progesterone is made initially by the corpus luteum (the sac in the ovary from which an egg has been released) during the latter half of the menstrual cycle. Small amounts are also produced in the adrenal glands. It is made from cholesterol, which is produced from the carbohydrates and fats we eat. Eating the right balance of these is therefore important. If a woman becomes pregnant, the corpus luteum continues to make progesterone to support the growing fetus until the placenta is mature enough to take over production.

Progesterone helps maintain an even weight by assisting the control of water retention and by promoting efficient thyroid function. It also helps the body use fat for energy.

For progesterone to do its job as part of the monthly cycle it has to get inside the cells of the uterus. It travels from the ovary in the blood; once inside the cell it is taken by a receptor to the nucleus which contains the instructions that enable it to support the fertilized ovum. Progesterone makes the uterine lining secrete food for the developing embryo and suppresses any immune rejection of the baby. If a progesterone receptor is not available to bind to it, it simply leaves the cell. As the menopause approaches, the number of progesterone receptors declines, reducing the chances of a successful pregnancy.

THE FATE OF ESTROGEN AND PROGESTERONE

After estrogen and progesterone have completed their tasks, they are taken in the blood to the liver, where they are deactivated and passed to the digestive tract for elimination. This constant production and breakdown, in response to the body's continual needs, is what controls the balance of hormones. An optimum supply of nutrients, including some B vitamins, helps ensure that the process runs smoothly. Research back in 1942, and more recently in the 1980s, has shown that low levels of magnesium may reduce the liver's ability to deactivate estrogen;[1] a deficiency of vitamin B6, which works alongside magnesium, has the same effect. B vitamin deficiencies were found as early as 1943 in women suffering from heavy periods and cystic mastitis. Treatment with less than 100mg a day brought about a dramatic reduction in symptoms.[2]

Adequate soluble fiber in the diet helps to bind sex hormones excreted into the digestive tract, aiding their elimination. Too little encourages their reactivation and reabsorption into circulation. Soluble fibers, such as fructo-oligosaccharides (FOS), selectively stimulate the beneficial bacteria in the gut known as bifido bacteria. A beneficial balance of these inhibits an enzyme that is capable of reactivating estrogen. FOS is present in small quantities in the diet and is available as a supplement.

Researchers have also found a direct link between the quantity of plant fiber eaten and the presence of a carrier molecule for estrogen in the blood called serum hormone binding globulin (SHBG).[3] Although still contested, there is now sufficient data to suggest that a diet rich in dietary fiber correlates positively with a high SHBG. The more SHBG is produced, the less free estrogen there is available to the estrogen–sensitive tissues.

SYNTHETIC HORMONES

We believe that it is virtually impossible for synthetic hormones to restore the natural hormone balance in the body: at best they can simulate the actions of natural hormones. In the last 30 years, synthetic varieties have been promoted as the answer to a whole spectrum of women's health problems, but there are more natural ways to balance hormones. We believe that women would not take the risk of using synthetic hormones if they knew the implications for their own health, that of their offspring, and ultimately for the future health of humanity, especially alongside exposure to environmental estrogen–like substances.

Sex hormones, natural or synthetic, are potent substances that have widespread effects. Synthetic forms of estrogen and progesterone (progestogens) are commonly prescribed. They are very similar in structure to natural hormones: the body accepts and uses them. However, although they bind with the same receptor sites in target cells, they may convey a different message. In addition, synthetic hormones are not so easily adjusted or disposed of by the body (their effectiveness is partly due to their ability to act in the body for longer than natural hormones). The two most popular forms of synthetic hormones are in the contraceptive pill and HRT (used as a "cure" for the menopause). However, these uses are not without their problems, as the next chapter explains.

....

CHAPTER 19

THE PILL AND HRT – EXPLODING THE MYTHS

With hindsight, it is likely that history will record the widespread prescribing of synthetic hormones to women as one of medicine's biggest ever bungles. Many women taking the contraceptive pill and HRT have little idea what they contain or how they act. Whatever the purpose of these treatments, their effect is to totally disrupt the natural balance and interaction of estrogen and progesterone in the body.

THE CONTRACEPTIVE PILL

Controlling fertility has been a major preoccupation for a long time. Back in the 1960s the time was ripe for effective contraception. Venereal diseases were being treated effectively, and constraining religious beliefs were being eroded. There was no longer the same social pressure to regulate women's sexuality. The market expanded rapidly, filling the coffers of the pharmaceutical industry.

One of the myths about the contraceptive pill is that it is a problem-free form of contraception. However, one early researcher, Dr Ellen Grant, author of *The Bitter Pill*, was shocked when synthetic hormones were not withdrawn from the market due to their known serious side-effects. The Pill is certainly a highly effective contraceptive, but it also creates problems, including: depletion of many vital nutrients; difficulty for some women in re-establishing a normal menstrual cycle or conceiving after stopping the Pill; raised blood pressure; risk of fatal blood clots; and a higher risk of certain types of cancer.

How the Pill Works

The Pill works by suppressing a woman's natural hormones, interfering with the natural balance of estrogen and progesterone. The production of luteinizing hormone (LH) is inhibited, preventing ovulation; cervical mucus becomes hostile to sperm; the lining of the uterus is altered so an egg has difficulty embedding in it; and the hormonal state of pregnancy is simulated. The Pill stops proper menstruation; bleeding – better termed withdrawal bleeding – only occurs each month when hormones are not taken for seven days.

How the Pill is Made

The hormones in contraceptive pills are made in pharmaceutical laboratories. Progestogens are most commonly manufactured from natural progesterone-like substances found in foods like soya and wild yam.

Known Risks of the Pill

The risks are similar for both the combined and the mini Pill. The combined Pill – a combination of synthetic estrogen and progestogen – is considered to be more potent. It should not be given to women who have ever suffered from blood clots, liver disease, high blood pressure, obesity, known or suspected breast or any other hormone-related cancers, or vaginal bleeding of unknown cause. Taking the combined Pill increases the risk of coronary artery disease, particularly in women who smoke. Some women with a history of epilepsy, migraine, asthma or heart disease find their symptoms get worse while taking the Pill. Changes in brain wave patterns (EEG) are seen in up to 60 per cent of women taking the combined Pill.

A woman should stop the mini Pill (which only contains progestogen) if she experiences any visual problems, headaches or migraines, or if she has any serious unexplained illness. Progestogen-only pills are sometimes recommended for women who have problems with the combined Pill.

It is advisable to contact your doctor immediately if any of the following occur: blood in the urine, dizziness or nose bleeds, fainting, migraines or unusually severe headaches, numbness or tingling, pregnancy, severe or sudden chest pain, coughing up blood, visual disturbance, yellowing of the skin.

Side-effects of the Pill

nausea, vomiting, headache, breast tenderness, weight changes, changes in sex drive, depression, blood clots, changes in skin color, high blood pressure, loss of periods, irregular bleeding

---

It should be understood that, although rarely, the Pill (particularly the combined Pill) can be life-threatening. It can lead to a fatal blood clot that ultimately blocks the blood supply in the lungs. Studies in Britain indicate that a woman who is on the Pill is twice as likely to experience a fatal blood clot as a non-Pill user.[4] The problem is so worrying that the Family Planning Association launched a public education campaign targeting Britain's three million Pill users.

Lesser Known Risks of the Pill

Synthetic hormones can affect the way the body uses many nutrients. The balance of these in the body is essential to ensure the precise synchrony of hormones as well as for countless other functions.

Vitamin A

Excessive levels of vitamin A have been found in the blood of women on the Pill. Supplementing vitamin A is not advisable while taking the Pill but it is important to ensure a good dietary intake. After stopping the Pill, however, supplementing vitamin A is important: the Pill elevates blood levels of the vitamin by mobilizing reserves in the liver, so stores need replenishing. The high level of vitamin A found in the blood of Pill users may partly explain why it helps skin problems like acne, and why stopping the Pill often brings about skin problems even in women who had not suffered from them before.

Vitamin C

Concern that vitamin C increases the potency of estrogen, by raising estradiol in the blood, led one group of researchers to caution Pill users against taking vitamin C supplements. A thorough investigation into such processes showed, however, that taking 1g of vitamin C daily does not raise estrogen levels in women on the Pill.[5] Even if vitamin C did strengthen estrogen, the body would compensate by producing less.

B Vitamins

Synthetic hormones are harder for the body to break down and eliminate. B vitamins – including choline and inositol – are involved in these processes in the liver, so it is wise to supplement extra B complex.

Vitamin K

While using the Pill, supplementing vitamin K (which is rarely included in multivitamins) should be avoided, as it is involved in blood clotting (and the risk of blood clots is increased by synthetic hormones). Dietary intake of vitamin K from green vegetables and cauliflower should not, however, be restricted.

Copper, Zinc, Manganese and Iron

Higher levels of copper are associated with Pill use. Since copper increases the amount of estrogen in the body, high copper levels may increase the risks associated with estrogen dominance. Copper also competes with zinc, which is required at every step of the reproductive process. It is best not to supplement copper unless supplementing ten times as much zinc. Too much zinc can also deplete iron and manganese, but, as Pill-takers usually lose less blood at the monthly bleed than in normal menstruation, extra iron supplementation may not be needed. Unless tests show an iron deficiency, taking more than the 10mg of iron found in a good multivitamin should not be necessary. For manganese, 3–5mg is sufficient. So an ideal mineral supplement might provide 15mg of zinc, 10mg of iron, 3mg of manganese and 1.5mg or less of copper.

Reduced Effectiveness

Some combined Pills are taken for 21 days, followed by a seven-day break. Other preparations are taken every day, and include a week's hormoneless pills. Daily use minimizes the risk of forgetting, thereby increasing reliability. Effectiveness can, however, be reduced by diarrhea and vomiting, and some medications, including antibiotics, sedatives, anti-arthritic drugs and anti-epileptic drugs.

The mini Pill must be taken every day, at the same time, to

maintain good contraceptive cover. A delay of only three hours can result in a loss of protection. Its effectiveness is high, but lower than that of the combined Pill.

HORMONE REPLACEMENT THERAPY (HRT)

Despite research showing the downside of HRT, it has been described as the most important preventive medicine of the century. Between 1963 and 1973 sales of estrogen preparations quadrupled and half the post-menopausal female population of Britain was using HRT.

According to the Amarant Trust, a charity that uncritically promotes HRT, the menopause is a "deficiency disease." By definition, diseases need to be treated, which is where HRT comes in. HRT has been recommended to prolong women's active sex lives after the menopause, and ever since its introduction figures have been manipulated to infer a variety of benefits, including stronger bones and protection from heart disease.

HRT is available in pills, patches and implants. Choosing the most appropriate form – from around 50 preparations – is not straightforward and is assessed largely according to risk and convenience. Some women take several years to find one that suits them. Some never find the right one. Surveys report that 70 per cent of women discontinue HRT within a year and only 7 per cent last eight years.[6]

The myth about HRT is that it is a "complete cure" for the menopause. It regularly relieves symptoms such as hot flashes, vaginal dryness and loss of libido but is considered by many to cause several other problems. HRT is said to prevent osteoporosis, protect against the risk of heart disease and lower blood pressure. But these claims have not been convincingly proven. Many studies report that HRT increases the risk of both breast and endometrial cancer;[7] it has not been in use long enough to determine its long-term effects on health.

How HRT Works

HRT – originally called "estrogen replacement therapy" – works by replacing the depleted estrogen levels that occur at the menopause. It is thought that low levels are responsible for the increased risk of heart disease and osteoporosis as well as many of the symptoms of menopause, including hot flashes, vaginal dryness and depression. The estrogen-only preparations were, however, soon linked to an increased risk of endometrial cancer and are no longer recommended for women who still have their uteri. Such women are prescribed a combination synthetic progestogen/estrogen treatment.

How HRT is Made

Unlike the Pill which mainly uses the synthetic estrogen, ethynylestradiol, most estrogens used in HRT are so-called "natural" i.e. taken from a pregnant mare's urine or the ovaries of pigs. Marilyn Glenville writes in her book *Natural Alternatives to HRT*, "Not all the estrogens in the mixture are natural to humans and some can behave like ethynlyestradiol, the synthetic hormone, which tends to affect liver metabolism by producing changes in blood clotting and blood fat levels." An official investigation by a representative of the World Society for the Protection of Animals reported that the mares were not kept in acceptable conditions. The synthetic progestogen used in HRT is the same as that in contraceptive pills.

Known Risks of HRT

Generally, the side-effects of HRT are similar to those associated with taking the Pill (see page 129). Taking estrogens by mouth is associated with nausea, vomiting, bloating and abdominal cramps. Oral estrogens go to the liver first to be broken down, so it is difficult to know how much will end up in the blood.

The skin patch bypasses the liver, giving a higher level of estrogen in the blood, and is associated with a localized discoloration of the skin.

Increasingly popular are estrogen implants: pellets are inserted under the skin in a small operation. They should last six months but frequently women return three to nine weeks later, complaining of recurring menopausal symptoms.[8] Implants are associated with an addiction to estrogen and it has been suggested that women who gain such tolerance to estrogen have psychiatric problems and require larger than normal amounts of estrogen!

Professor Howard Jacobs, of the Middlesex Hospital in London, suggests that it may be the continual saturation of the estrogen-sensitive cells that makes them lose the ability to respond accordingly. It is also indicated that early use of estrogen, in the Pill, may set the stage for an increased need for replacement therapy.

For two years after stopping estrogen implants, there is still a risk of developing endometrial cancer. To lower the risk, a woman needs to take a progestogen for two years or more after discontinuing an estrogen implant.

....

CHAPTER 20

THE PROGESTERONE STORY

Progesterone literally means necessary "for pregnancy" (pro-gestation). In 1929, three years after estrogen had been identified in the urine of menstruating women, progesterone was identified in the corpus luteum. Modern science now enables us not only to identify hormones but to begin to understand how they exert their influence in the body.

WHERE DOES PROGESTERONE COME FROM?

Several years after progesterone was identified, it was realized that large amounts were also produced in the placenta, and human placentas were soon the major source of progesterone used in experimental work. In 1939 it was found that sapogenin, in the sarsaparilla plant, could be converted into a progesterone-like compound. Soon afterwards diosgenin, a substance in wild yam, was converted in the laboratory into progesterone, in exactly the same form as the body produces.

By the early 1950s, thousands of plants were found to contain active estrogen and progesterone-like substances called phyto-estrogens and phyto-progesterones. (see Chapter 24 for more information on phytonutrients/hormones). The major modern source of diosgenin is the soya bean. The body cannot convert diosgenin into progesterone itself.

It is possible to produce not only synthetic forms of

progesterone (progestogens) but also estrogen and the male hormone testosterone. The manufacture of altered forms is easy and cheap and, because they are not natural, they can be patented for great profit. Despite early and continued success by some physicians using progesterone for PMS, threatened miscarriage and ovarian cysts, research into natural hormones declined, in the face of competition from synthetic forms.

Progesterone is the only hormone in the body produced in milligrams. All others are produced in nanogram amounts. By the last three months of pregnancy the body produces up to 30 times more than it does in the non-pregnant state. Progesterone is not gender-specific: baby boys do not turn into baby girls under the influence of progesterone.

What does progesterone do?

Progesterone maintains a lush endometrium, ensuring that the developing baby is well nourished throughout pregnancy. When it is first produced, following ovulation, a woman's sex drive is at its height. Progesterone plays a pivotal role in the synchrony of other steroid hormones: the body uses it to make the three major estrogens, testosterone, the stress hormone cortisol and other corticosteroids, plus aldosterone (which helps control water balance in the body). Progesterone's production and conversion into other hormones is critical for hormone balance.

It has a variety of other important biological effects. It helps:

- the body use fat for energy
- lift mood by acting as a natural anti-depressant
- the thyroid hormones work properly, assisting weight control
- prevent the blood from clotting inappropriately
- keep the correct balance of zinc and copper in the body

- the cells in the body maintain proper oxygen levels (an important factor in the prevention of cancer)
- protect against fibrocystic breast disease and breast cancer
- protect against endometrial cancer
- redress the harmful effects of too much estrogen

Synthetic progesterone – progestogens – are not capable of matching the full range of progesterone's functions. However, they fit the progesterone receptor sites, blocking the ability of the natural hormone to carry out its functions. Because progestogens are stronger and more potent, they are also more difficult for the body to de-activate and break down.

So, even if the body is producing enough progesterone, it may not be able to exert its influence if synthetic hormones get in the way. Similarly, xenoestrogens (the estrogen mimics used by the chemical and agricultural industries) can block the action of the natural hormone and scramble the message.

DO WE HAVE A SHORTAGE OF PROGESTERONE?

For hormones to work well, they need to be in balance. In modern times this appears to be a difficult condition to fulfil. The insidious competition from synthetic hormones (mainly estrogens), xenoestrogens and those fed to animals to fatten them up is often too much of a challenge for the body to deal with by producing more progesterone. Exposure to xenoestrogens can directly inhibit the body's ability to produce progesterone.

In addition to this, women become estrogen dominant from their mid-thirties onwards, as they increasingly do not ovulate with every menstrual cycle. Some doctors believe that anovulatory cycles are epidemic among women in industrialized countries.

The effect of not ovulating with each cycle is that no

progesterone is produced and the body is exposed to estrogen only throughout the month (see Fig. 6). Sub-optimum nutrition, stress and too much exercise are believed to contribute to anovulatory cycles. However, it is xenoestrogen exposure that is considered to be the most potent factor involved. It is often possible to detect an anovulatory period due to a change in pattern and heavier, longer or shorter periods.

Due to the regular occurrence of anovulatory cycles before the menopause, estrogen levels become increasingly dominant. This can lead to the exaggerated symptoms of too much estrogen experienced before the menopause. This is compounded by the fact that the pituitary gland is instructed to release high levels of follicle stimulating hormone (FSH) and luteinizing hormone (LH) in response to a low level of progesterone, which can lead to an increased production of estrogens.

Even ovulatory cycles can lead to estrogen dominance if

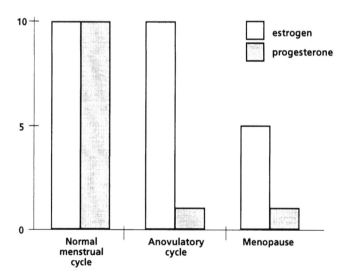

Figure 6 – Estrogen and progesterone ratios

they are either too short or too long; the first half of the cycle is normally 14 days but can last up to six weeks or more. The second half of the cycle is more constant – usually between 10 and 16 days. Estrogen dominance is more likely to arise in the second half of an ovulatory cycle as progesterone is around for a shorter period of time in relation to estrogen.

PROBLEMS ASSOCIATED WITH ESTROGEN DOMINANCE IN WOMEN

Breast cancer is strongly associated with too much estrogen. The most common time for breast cancer to develop is five years before the menopause when estrogen dominance is likely to be highest due to anovulatory cycles.

Endometrial cancer of the lining of the uterus has only one known cause – unopposed estrogen.

PMS is strongly associated with hormonal imbalance. It produces a multitude of symptoms that often appear diverse and unrelated but which are similar to those associated with too much estrogen.

An underactive thyroid gland can give rise to a similar set of symptoms to estrogen dominance and PMS. Too much estrogen affects the thyroid hormone.

Blood sugar levels are affected by the presence of too much estrogen. Symptoms are similar to estrogen dominance, PMS and thyroid problems. The hormones insulin and glucagon and the stress hormone cortisol are all involved in the control of blood sugar levels. Stress hormones are made from progesterone in the body, so low levels can adversely affect the way we cope with stress.

Other Health Problems Associated with Estrogen Dominance

rapid aging, allergies, breast tenderness, depression, fatigue, fibrocystic breast disease, fibroids, headaches, infertility, irritability, memory loss, miscarriage, osteoporosis, reduced sex drive, water retention

---

WHAT HAPPENS WHEN PROGESTERONE LEVELS DECREASE?

Low progesterone levels can increase estrogen through the production of another hormone called androstenedione. When progesterone levels fall, either as a result of anovulatory cycles or post-menopausally, the body responds by increasing the production of androstenedione, a masculinizing hormone which is one step in a pathway for making estrogen. (Men make most of their estrogen from this hormone.) After the menopause, androstenedione and a similar masculinizing hormone called androstenediol become the major producers of estrogen in the body.

Cholesterol is converted to a hormone called pregnenolone which is either made into progesterone or another hormone called DHEA (dihydroepiandrosterone). From DHEA, the body is able to make androstenedione or androstenediol, either of which can be converted into testosterone or estrogens (see Fig. 7). If estrogen is made this way, there is a tendency (particularly if the receptor sites for estrogen are filled with synthetic or xenoestrogens) for testosterone to be formed instead. This can lead to symptoms like hair loss on the scalp and unwanted hair on the legs and face.

At menopause, the production of estrogen in the body only falls by half to one-third. Progesterone decreases to 120th of baseline levels, yet it is estrogen that is widely prescribed to

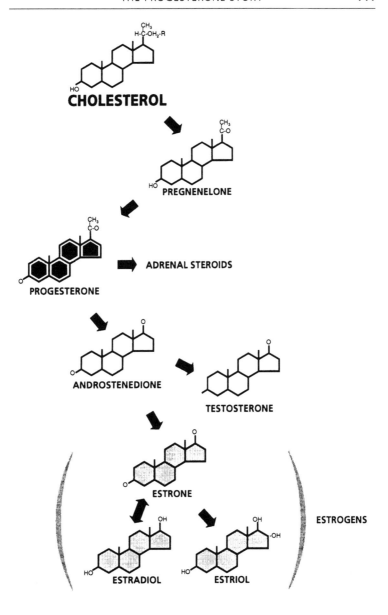

Figure 7 – How hormones are made from cholesterol

treat menopausal symptoms and protect against osteoporosis and heart disease. With environmental and synthetic hormone exposure too, it is little wonder that progesterone has a hard task keeping estrogen in check.

REDRESSING THE BALANCE

It is important to realize that estrogen is a vital hormone for human survival. It is the imbalance of estrogen to progesterone, and not excess estrogen per se, that is thought to be responsible for many of today's female health problems.

Fifty years ago, when man-made chemicals were first used in industry, little thought was given to their potential effects on reproduction. More concern at that time was focused on whether they were likely to be carcinogenic (cancer-forming). Only now are we realizing that the by-products of man-made, industrial chemicals are capable of wreaking havoc with hormone balance in all species.

We are unlikely ever to understand the complexity of hormonal interaction in its entirety but the measures for maintaining and improving health described in this book are sound in regard to the perceived problem. In redressing the balance between estrogen and progesterone (for those that have accepted that the problem exists), there are two possible approaches:

1 Ensure optimum nutrient intake and the healthiest possible lifestyle, including reduced exposure to pollutants.

2 As 1, plus, where necessary, the use of progesterone applied to the skin, derived from soya or wild yam, at levels the body would produce for itself (see Chapter 21).

It is clear that optimum nutrition and a sensible lifestyle are key components in addressing the problem of estrogen dominance. Part 5 gives a full account of how you can optimize your nutrient intake.

NATURAL HORMONES – THE SAFE ALTERNATIVE

Natural hormones are essential substances that help to keep us fit and healthy when they are in balance. Cells all over the body recognize natural hormones – they fit like hand in glove – and therefore respond to them appropriately.

Progesterone is a key hormone from which estrogens are made; and almost everything in the body is ultimately made from the food we eat. To make nature's hormones work best, it is therefore sensible to provide your body with the best possible raw materials. Part 5 of this book shows you how to do this.

Addressing the problem of estrogen dominance through an optimum diet and lifestyle alone may, however, not be enough for some women. In certain instances, we believe it is appropriate to replace a deficient hormone with one derived from a natural source such as soya or wild yam, that has been converted in the laboratory to exactly the same structure as the body would have made for itself.

Where an actual disease associated with estrogen dominance has already been diagnosed, such as fibroids, fibrocystic breasts or osteoporosis, then the case for supplementing a naturally derived hormone is even stronger. Combining natural hormone supplements with an optimized diet and lifestyle should increase the chances of such health problems responding well.

There is no conclusive evidence so far that shows that an optimum diet alone will significantly reverse the process of osteoporosis. However, Dr John Lee has demonstrated, over two decades of clinical practice, an increase in bone density of up to 15 per cent in three years, using a natural transdermal cream (applied to the skin) containing progesterone.

SUPPLEMENTING NATURAL PROGESTERONE

Natural progesterone, as found in transdermal creams such as Progest, has minimal, transient side-effects if taken as recommended. Some women report temporary, incidental spotting in the first three months of use. Any persistent spotting or breakthrough bleeding should be reported to your doctor; likewise, if you experience headaches or other progressive symptoms.

During the first few months of use, symptoms of estrogen dominance, including breast tenderness, breast swelling and weight gain, may be exaggerated. This is because estrogen and progesterone are closely interrelated, and, although they generally oppose one other, each helps the other by making target organ cells more sensitive. In time, however, when sufficient progesterone has been absorbed through the fatty layers of the skin, this effect should stop.

The ability of estrogen and progesterone to make the cells of a target organ more sensitive has given cause for concern because, during the first three months of use, progesterone could in fact promote a cancer by stimulating estrogen-sensitive target organs like the breast or uterus.

Indeed, several studies have indicated that progesterone is carcinogenic, but under closer scrutiny they either refer to a progestogen (synthetic progesterone) or the levels of progesterone used have been well above any level that the body would naturally produce. For example, in one study a strain of rats known to be prone to developing cancer were given a cancer-promoting agent and excessively high levels of progesterone to see if giving progesterone would speed up the process, which it did. This study was mercilessly criticized for its methodology at the time, but it is still used by some to support a case for progesterone being carcinogenic.

Similarly, it has been claimed that progesterone suppresses the immune system. Undoubtedly, progesterone has a localized immuno-suppressive effect in the uterus during pregnancy to prevent any immune rejection of the baby which contains its father's "foreign" proteins. However, research generally indicates that, during pregnancy, the overall effect of the increased production of progesterone is to enhance the function of the immune system.[9]

Recent research (as described on page 92) indicates that progesterone is protective to breast tissue. Dr John Lee's hypothesizes:

> When estrogen and progesterone receptor testing of breast cancer cells is done, it is generally the rule that progesterone receptors are not found unless plenty of estrogen receptors are present. Estrogen stimulates the emergence of progesterone receptors. Since estrogen stimulates cell proliferation (which is not desirable in cancer cells) and progesterone inhibits proliferation in favor of cell maturation, it would seem wise to supply the needed progesterone.

It has been our experience that, in a minority of women, symptoms of breast tenderness, breast swelling and weight gain do not respond to progesterone creams well, even after six months of use. Many more do, however, especially when combined with optimum nutrition. The reasons for this are unclear. One suggestion is that some women do not absorb progesterone efficiently through the skin into the bloodstream, accumulating it in the skin instead.

If you take thyroid medication, consult your medical practitioner because progesterone increases thyroid activity, so you may require a lower dose of medication.

SUPPLEMENTING NATURAL ESTROGEN

In some instances, Dr John Lee has found that supplementing a natural source of estrogen has been necessary to manage resistant hot flashes and vaginal dryness. However, estrogen supplementation is not advisable for women with diabetes, varicose veins, a high blood fat level, high blood pressure, fibrocystic breasts, fibroids, obesity, a history of breast cancer, endometrial cancer, ovarian cancer or any clotting disorders.

TESTING YOUR HORMONE LEVELS

We believe that the best way to identify whether you would benefit from progesterone is to have your hormone levels checked, usually by a blood test. A more sensitive test involves taking a simple saliva sample, this reveals the amount of free circulating hormone, which is the best indicator not only of progesterone levels but also of other hormones including the three main estrogens, testosterone and DHEA. If you are using a natural hormone cream, it is wise to have your levels tested annually.

Most ION-trained nutritionists or a nutritionally orientated doctor could recommend saliva or blood hormone tests.

Hormones, natural or otherwise, should be used with care and are only available on prescription in Britain. Many natural hormones are available over the counter in the USA and some other countries but we do not recommend that you self-prescribe them. A nutritionist can work with you to optimize your diet and lifestyle, and recommend appropriate tests. If your own GP is unwilling to prescribe a natural hormone for you, a list of medically qualified practitioners who will is available from Higher Nature. By calling the Natural Progesterone Information Line you can request information on natural progesterone to be sent to yourself and your GP.

CHAPTER 22

NATURAL HORMONES – HOW AND WHEN TO USE THEM

The subject of how and when to use natural estrogen cream and DHEA is too complex for the confines of this book. However, natural estrogen cream has been used successfully to help manage hot flashes and vaginal dryness in some women where natural progesterone alone proved insufficient. DHEA has been used to help manage weight problems, immune problems and stress. We strongly recommend that you only consider natural hormone supplementation under the guidance of a medical practitioner familiar with their use and a nutritionist who can optimize your diet and lifestyle.

USING NATURAL PROGESTERONE

Massage progesterone cream into the skin until it becomes well absorbed. The cream can be applied to any area of the body, but is best absorbed where the skin is thinner – in places such as the neck, chest, breast, lower abdomen, inner thighs, wrists, palms and inner arms. Regularly rotate the application of the cream to different parts of the body for maximum effect and to reduce any localized reaction to the cream. A few women have reacted to some added component to the cream.

Natural progesterone is available as a cream in a 50g (2 oz) tube or in a 25ml (1 fl oz) bottle. The oil and the cream can be used together for the management of persistent menopausal problems like hot flashes. Natural progesterone oil can be taken directly under the tongue or, if you don't like the taste, it can be rubbed into the soles of the feet. If you use this method, apply the oil at night and wear old socks to prevent staining the bed clothes.

Pre-menstrual Syndrome (PMS)

Natural progesterone cream can help reduce symptoms associated with PMS. The cream is used in a way that would simulate the natural menstrual cycle (see Fig. 8). Read Chapter 8 for further guidance on PMS.

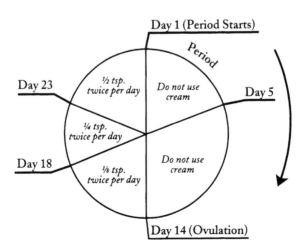

Figure 8 – Pre-menstrual

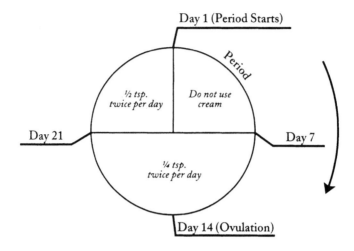

Figure 9 – Menopause

Menopause

Women respond to the menopause differently, some with mild and some with acute symptoms, so each one's requirements for progesterone will vary. Start with the guidelines given here and adjust the level to meet your needs. If you have stopped menstruating, use the same schedule but base it on the calendar month (see Fig. 9).

Persistent Vaginal Dryness and Hot Flashes

Natural progesterone cream, used vaginally, has been very successful in treating vaginal dryness – insert a quarter to half a teaspoon daily in addition to your usual application.

For hot flashes use extra natural progesterone cream for immediate relief of symptoms – a quarter to half a teaspoon every 15 minutes for one hour following the hot flash.

For persistent menopausal symptoms, progesterone oil is more effective. For hot flashes, place 2–5 drops of the oil under the tongue and retain it for five minutes. Repeat the dose every 10–15 minutes for the hour after the hot flash. The oil may also be rubbed into the soles of your feet. Chapter 11 gives more advice on dealing with menopause.

Osteoporosis

It is a good idea to determine the extent of your bone loss before starting treatment with natural progesterone cream and then check yearly whether the situation has improved. If you have severe osteoporosis or have experienced fractures, then double the dose of progesterone cream over the same time-span (Fig. 10). Chapter 12 gives further guidance on treating osteoporosis.

Natural progesterone can also be helpful for a range of other health problems, some of which are discussed in Part 3.

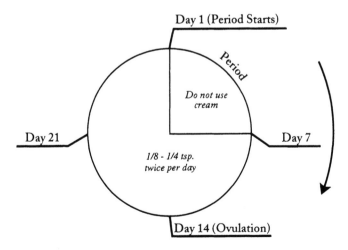

Figure 10 – Osteoporosis

PART 5

ACTION PLAN FOR HORMONAL HEALTH

CHAPTER 23

Diet for the Good Life

The perfect diet is one that provides every single cell in the body with the best supply of nutrients – it is the foundation of health. If we examine the diets of other cultures renowned for living to a ripe old age, it is clear such people eat a varied and natural diet.

The Diet for the Good Life aims to give you maximum hormonal health; when your hormones are balanced and healthy then the rest of your body should be healthy too. The basis of this diet is plenty of complex carbohydrates, moderate amounts of protein, sufficient essential fats, a minimum of saturated fats and plenty of water. The foods recommended also provide an alkaline-forming diet and give you good levels of vitamins and minerals, both consistent with optimal health. For more detailed advice on following a perfect diet, we suggest you consult *The Optimum Nutrition Bible* (see Recommended Reading).

FATS

There are two kinds of fat: saturated (hard) fat, and unsaturated fat. It is not essential to eat saturated fat, nor is it advisable to eat too much. The main sources are meat and dairy products. There are also two kinds of unsaturated fats: monounsaturated, of which olive oil is a rich source;

and polyunsaturated fats, found in nut and seed oils and fish.

Certain polyunsaturated fats, called linoleic and linolenic acid or Omega 6 and Omega 3 oils, are vital for the brain and nervous system, immune system, cardiovascular system and skin. A common sign of deficiency of these substances is dry skin. The optimal diet provides a balance of these two essential fats. Pumpkin and flax seeds are rich in linolenic acid (Omega 3), while sesame and sunflower seeds are rich in linoleic acid (Omega 6). Linolenic acid is converted in the body into DHA and EPA, which are also found in mackerel, herring, salmon and tuna. These essential fats are easily destroyed by heating or exposure to oxygen, so it is important to have a fresh daily source and not to use them for cooking.

The ideal mix is one half flax seed, the other half equal portions of pumpkin, sunflower and sesame, kept unground in the fridge, in a sealed glass container, and ground on the day for use.

Processed foods often contain hardened or hydrogenated polyunsaturated fats. These are worse for you than saturated fat and are best avoided.

- **Eat** 1 tablespoon cold-pressed seed oil (sesame, sunflower, pumpkin, flax seed, etc) or 1 heaped tablespoon mixed ground seeds a day.

- **Avoid** fried food, burnt or browned fat, saturated and hydrogenated fat.

Protein

The 25 amino acids (components of protein) are the building blocks of the body. As well as being vital for growth and the repair of body tissue, they are used to make hormones, enzymes, antibodies and neurotransmitters, and help transport substances around the body. Both the quality of the protein you eat (determined by the balance of these amino acids), and the quantity you eat, are important.

The government recommends that we obtain 15 per cent of our total calorie intake from protein, but gives little guidance as to the kind of protein we should choose. This is in sharp contrast to the average breast-fed baby who receives just 1 per cent of its total calories from protein and manages to double its birth weight in six months. This is because the protein from breast milk is very good quality and easily absorbed. Assuming good-quality protein, 10 per cent of calorie intake, or around 40g of protein a day, is an optimal intake for most people, unless pregnant, recovering from surgery, or undertaking large amounts of exercise or heavy manual work.

The best-quality protein foods, in terms of amino acid balance, include eggs, quinoa (a grain that cooks like rice), soya, meat, fish, beans and lentils. Animal protein sources tend to contain a lot of undesirable saturated fat, whereas vegetable protein sources tend to contain additional beneficial complex carbohydrates and are less acid-forming than meat. It is best to limit meat to three meals a week. It is difficult not to take in adequate protein from any diet that includes three meals a day, whether you are vegan, vegetarian or meat-eating. Many vegetables, especially seed foods like runner beans, peas, corn or broccoli, contain good levels of protein and help to neutralize excess acidity which can lead to loss of minerals including calcium (hence the higher risk of osteoporosis among frequent meat-eaters).

- **Eat** two servings of beans, lentils, quinoa, tofu (soya), seed vegetables or other vegetable protein, or one small serving of meat, fish, cheese, or a free-range egg.

- **Avoid** excess animal protein.

CARBOHYDRATES

Carbohydrate is the main fuel for the body. It comes in two forms: fast-releasing, as in sugar, honey, malt, sweets and most refined foods; and slow-releasing, as in wholegrains, vegetables and fresh fruit. The latter foods contain more complex carbohydrate and/or more fiber, both of which help to slow down the release of sugar. Fast-releasing carbohydrates tend to give a sudden burst of energy, followed by a slump, while slow-releasing carbohydrates provide more sustained energy and are therefore preferable. Refined foods, like sugar or white flour, lack the vitamins and minerals needed for the body to use them properly and are best avoided. The constant use of fast-releasing carbohydrates can give rise to complex symptoms and health problems. Some fruit, like bananas, dates and raisins, contain faster-releasing sugars and are best kept to a minimum by people with glucose-related health problems. Slow-releasing carbohydrate foods – fresh fruit, vegetables, pulses and wholegrains – should make up two-thirds of what you eat, or around 70 per cent of your total calorie intake.

- **Eat** five servings of raw or lightly cooked dark green, leafy and root vegetables such as watercress, carrots, sweet potatoes, broccoli, Brussels sprouts, spinach, green beans or peppers.

- **Eat** three or more servings of fresh fruit such as apples, pears, berries, melon or citrus fruit.

- **Eat** four or more servings of wholegrains such as brown rice, millet, rye, oats, wholewheat, corn, quinoa, breads, pasta or pulses.

- **Avoid** any form of sugar, foods with added sugar, white or refined foods.

FIBER

Rural Africans eat about 55g of dietary fiber a day (compared to the UK average intake of 22g and have among the lowest incidence in the world of bowel diseases such as appendicitis, diverticulitis, colitis and bowel cancer. The ideal intake is not less than 35g a day. It is easy to get this amount of fiber – which absorbs water in the digestive tract, making the food contents bulkier and easier to pass through the body – by eating wholegrains, vegetables, fruit, nuts, seeds, lentils and beans on a daily basis. Fruit and vegetable fiber slows down the absorption of sugar into the blood, helping to maintain good energy levels. Cereal fiber is particularly important in preventing constipation and putrefaction of foods, which are underlying causes of many digestive complaints. Refined diets that include a lot of meat, eggs, fish and dairy produce will undoubtedly lack fiber.

- **Eat** wholefoods – wholegrains, lentils, beans, nuts, seeds, fresh fruit and vegetables.

- **Avoid** refined, white and overcooked foods.

WATER

Two-thirds of the body consists of water, which is therefore our most important nutrient. The body loses about 1.5 liters (2½ pints) of water a day through the skin, lungs, gut and via the kidneys as urine, ensuring that toxic substances are eliminated from the body. We also make about 300ml (½ pint) of water a day when glucose is burned for energy. Therefore, the minimum water intake from food and drink is more than 1 liter (2 pints) a day, and the ideal intake is around 2 liters (4 pints) a day.

Fruit and vegetables consist of around 90 per cent water. They supply it in a form that is very easy for the body to use, at the same time providing the body with a high percentage of vitamins and minerals. Four pieces of fruit and four servings of vegetables, amounting to about 1.1kg (2¼ lb) of these foods, can provide 1 liter (2 pints) water, leaving a daily 1 liter

(2 pints) to be taken as water or in the form of diluted juices or herb or fruit teas. Alcohol, tea and coffee cause the body to lose water, so they are not recommended as sources of fluid intake. They also rob the body of valuable minerals.

- **Drink** 1 liter (2 pints) water a day as water or in diluted juices, herb or fruit teas

- **Minimize** your intake of alcohol, coffee, tea, and carbonated drinks

VITAMINS

Although vitamins are needed in much smaller amounts than fat, protein or carbohydrate, they are no less important. They "turn on" enzymes, which in turn make all body processes happen. Vitamins are needed to balance hormones, produce energy, boost the immune system, make healthy skin and protect the arteries; they are vital for the brain, nervous system and just about every physical process. Vitamins A, C and E are antioxidants – they slow down the aging process and protect the body from cancer, heart disease and pollution. B and C vitamins are vital for turning food into mental and physical energy. Vitamin D, found in milk, eggs, fish and meat, helps control calcium balance. It can also be made in the skin in the presence of sunshine; B and C vitamins are richest in living foods – fresh fruit and vegetables. Vitamin A comes in two forms: retinol, the animal form found in meat, fish, eggs and dairy produce; and beta-carotene, found in red, yellow and orange fruits and vegetables. Vitamin E is found in seeds, nuts and their oils and helps protect essential fats from going rancid.

- **Eat** three or more servings of dark green, leafy and root vegetables and three or more servings of fresh fruit, plus some nuts or seeds, every day.

- **Supplement** a multivitamin containing at least the following: 2250mcg vitamin A, 10mcg vitamin D, 100mg vitamin E, 25mg vitamin B1, 25mg B2, 50mg B3 (niacin), 50mg B5 (pantothenic acid), 50mg B6, 5mcg B12, 100mcg folic acid, 50mcg biotin. Also supplement 1000mg vitamin C a day.

Minerals

Like vitamins, minerals are essential for just about every process in the body. Calcium, magnesium and phosphorus help make up the bones and teeth. Nerve signals, vital for the brain and muscles, depend on calcium, magnesium, sodium and potassium. Oxygen is carried in the blood by an iron compound. Chromium helps control blood sugar levels. Zinc is vital for all body repair, renewal and development. Selenium and zinc help boost the immune system. Brain function depends on adequate magnesium, manganese, zinc and other essential minerals. These are but a few out of the thousands of key functions that minerals perform in human health.

We need large daily amounts of calcium and magnesium, which are found in vegetables such as kale, cabbage and root vegetables. They are also abundant in nuts and seeds. Calcium alone is found in large quantities in dairy produce. Fruits and vegetables also provide large amounts of potassium and small amounts of sodium, which is the right balance. All seed foods (which include seeds, nuts, lentils and beans, as well as peas, broad beans, runner beans, wholegrains and even broccoli (the heads are the seeds) are good sources of iron, zinc, manganese and chromium. Selenium is abundant in nuts, seafood, seaweed and seeds, especially sesame.

- **Eat** one serving of mineral-rich food such as kale, cabbage, root vegetables, low-fat dairy such as yoghurt, seeds or nuts such as almonds, as well as plenty of fresh fruit, vegetables and wholefoods such as lentils, beans and wholegrains.

- **Supplement** a multimineral containing at least the following: 150mg calcium, 75mg magnesium, 10mg iron, 10mg zinc, 2.5mg manganese, 50mcg chromium, 25mcg selenium.

PURE FOOD

Organic, unadulterated wholefoods have formed the basis of the human diet through the ages. Only now, in the twentieth century, has the human race been subjected to countless man-made chemicals in our food and our environment.

One major requirement for health is to eat foods that provide exactly the amount of energy required to keep the body in perfect balance. However, we waste a good deal of energy trying to disarm these alien and often toxic chemicals, some of which cannot be eliminated and end up accumulating in body tissue. It is now impossible to avoid all such substances, as there is nowhere on this planet that is not contaminated in some way by the products of our modern chemical age. So choosing organic foods whenever possible is the nearest we can get to eating a pure diet today. By supporting the movement back to producing these kinds of food we help to minimize the damage from chemical pollution which poses a real threat to the future of humanity.

Raw, organic food is the most natural and beneficial way to take food into the body. Many foods contain enzymes that help digest them once the food is chewed. Raw food is full of vital phytochemicals whose effect on our health may prove as important as vitamins and minerals. Cooking food destroys enzymes and reduces the activity of phytochemicals.

- **Eat** organic as much as you can. Make sure at least half your diet consists of raw fruit, vegetables, wholegrains, nuts and seeds.

- **Avoid** processed food containing lots of additives, and cook foods as little as possible.

Diet for the Good Life

Follow these 10 top tips daily for better health:

1 heaped tablespoon of ground seeds or 1 tablespoon of cold-pressed seed oil

2 servings of beans, lentils, quinoa, tofu (soya), or seed vegetables

3 pieces of fresh fruit such as apples, pears, berries, melon or citrus fruit

4 servings of wholegrains such as brown rice, millet, rye, oats, wholewheat, corn, quinoa as cereal, bread or pasta

5 servings of dark green, leafy and root vegetables such as watercress, carrots, sweet potatoes, broccoli, spinach, green beans, peas and peppers

6 glasses of water, diluted juices, herb or fruit teas

7 Eat whole, organic, raw food as much as possible

8 Supplement a high strength multivitamin and multi-mineral and 1000mg of vitamin C a day

9 Avoid fried, burnt, or browned food, hydrogenated fat and excess animal fat

10 Avoid any form of sugar as well as white, refined or processed food containing chemical additives, and minimize your intake of alcohol, coffee or tea – have no more than 1 unit of alcohol a day (e.g. a glass of wine, 300ml (½ pint) beer or lager, or 1 measure of a spirit).

CHAPTER 24

Phytonutrients – the Hormone Helpers

Hormone-like substances abound in natural foods. This is hardly surprising since hormones are, after all, made from food components. However, we have only recently recognized the extent to which foods that are rich in certain phytonutrients influence our hormone balance and health.

Phyto-estrogens – Friends or Foes?

Estrogen-like plant compounds are often called phyto-estrogens (phyto = plant). At first glance, given the health problems associated with estrogen dominance, one might think that eating foods rich in phyto-estrogens might be bad news. Yet the reverse seems to be true. Soya products, rich in the isoflavones genistein and daidzein, are reputed to protect against breast and prostate cancer, which are notably rare among communities with a soya-based diet.

Two possible explanations may explain this apparent contradiction. The first is that phyto-estrogens may lock onto and block the body's estrogen receptors, thereby making it harder for harmful chemicals to disrupt hormone signals. The second is that these phytonutrients may act more like hormone regulators, rather than simply mimicking estrogen or progesterone. Since mankind has been exposed to these plant chemicals for millennia, it is highly likely that our bodies have adapted to deal with them in the kind of quantities we are exposed to from eating natural foods.

While the general consensus is in favor of eating foods rich in these phytonutrients in moderate amounts, there are also grounds for caution, i.e. not giving vast amounts of phyto-estrogen rich foods, especially at key phases of development, such as during pregnancy or early infancy. (Some animals exclusively fed on soya feed have shown toxic effects.)

Nature's Hormone Helpers

Soya products and tofu are both excellent sources of isoflavones, which are powerful phyto-estrogens. Isoflavones are known to decrease the risk of hormone-related cancers, including breast and prostate cancer.[1] Two particular isoflavones have been identified – genistein and daidzein. An ideal intake is around 5mg a day, which is equivalent to a 350ml (12 fl oz) serving of soya milk or a 350g (12 oz) serving of tofu. Tofu, a curd made from the soya bean, is the richest source of isoflavones, while very processed soya products are the poorest source.[2]

Citrus fruits, wheat, alfalfa, hops, oats, fennel, celery and rhubarb all contain phyto-estrogens. There is a small amount of evidence that these foods may help to balance hormones and could play a part in part in helping to reduce symptoms associated with hormonal imbalance.[3]

Phytonutrient Herbal Remedies

Many herbal remedies are now available as supplements on the basis of their beneficial effects on hormone balance.

Agnus Castus

The plant Vitex Agnus Castus has a long history as a medicinal herb for women. Traditionally it has been used to relieve premenstrual and menopausal problems. One study of 1542 women using it found that 90 per cent reported a significant reduction of PMS symptoms.[4] Agnus Castus acts on the pituitary gland, mimicking the action of corpus luteum which produces progesterone. By stimulating the release of luteinizing hormone (LH), and inhibiting the release of follicle stimulating hormone (FSH), progesterone levels would tend to be increased in relation to estrogen.[5]

Black Cohosh, Dong Quai and Wild Yam

These all have progesterone-favorable effects on the body. Yams are especially rich in diosgenin, from which progesterone can be made in the laboratory. We cannot, however, turn these phytonutrients into progesterone itself. So, while these plants may help to balance hormones, they do not replace the need for progesterone in a person who is progesterone-deficient. Fennel also has a progesterone-favorable effect on hormone balance.

Ginseng and Licorice

These are considered to contain quite powerful adaptogens (substances that help restore hormonal balance). For example, licorice appears to strengthen estrogen when levels are too low and inhibit estrogen when levels are too high. Both licorice and ginseng influence adrenal hormones, responsible for stress. Ginseng is a classic herbal remedy for increasing one's ability to deal with stress. Both have widespread uses for a number of hormonal-related conditions probably because adrenal hormones and sex hormones are very closely related, with the adrenal glands producing small amounts of sex hormones.

Damiana and Saw Palmetto

These are probably the two most popular herbs for male hormonal health. Saw palmetto is best known for the treatment of prostatitis (enlargement of the prostate gland), a condition frequently suffered by men over 40. Damiana, which has a testosterone-like effect, has long been associated with increasing male potency.[5] These herbs, together with ginseng, are often included in male herbal tonics.

In summary, including the right phytonutrient foods and herbs in your diet may help your body to adapt, thus restoring and maintaining hormonal balance. Many supplements designed to support female or male health contain combinations of these herbs and are likely to be beneficial. However, large amounts of these herbs should only be taken under the guidance of a qualified nutrition consultant or herbalist.

....

CHAPTER 25

ESSENTIAL SUPPLEMENTS

The wealth of evidence supporting the value of nutritional supplements is substantial and we certainly recommend anyone seeking optimal hormonal health to consider taking them. The reason for supplementing is to guarantee that you are achieving optimal levels of every single nutrient that your body needs to maintain health and slow down the aging process. Due to modern intensive farming methods, food processing, the length of time food is stored and our exposure to toxins and pollutants a well-balanced diet will not provide optimum nutrition. We take supplements every day, and have seen them reverse profound hormonal problems and literally save people's lives.

Ideal levels vary from person to person: for maximum hormonal health we recommend you take the dosage levels shown in the chart overleaf, in addition to eating as good a diet as you can. We have listed the ideal levels for maintaining health and the levels required for therapeutic use for those with specific hormonal health problems. These correction levels are best taken under the advice and support of your doctor or a nutrition consultant. We advise pregnant women, and those women taking any form of regular medication to seek expert help.

We recommend you take these correction levels if the Hormonal Health Questionnaire on pages 42–44 indicated that you have a high risk for hormonal imbalances or if you suffer from PMS, menopausal symptoms, osteoporosis, fibrocystic breast disease, breast cancer, cervical dysplasia, fibroids, ovarian cysts or endometriosis. These levels are also appropriate if you are pregnant; do, however, make sure you don't supplement more than 7500iu of retinol (the animal form of vitamin A), as it has been shown to be toxic. Beta-carotene, the vegetable form of vitamin A, has no risk of toxicity.

If you are post-menopausal or have osteoporosis we also recommend you increase your intake of certain bone-building nutrients (If you are pregnant, breast-feeding or considering becoming pregnant than see page 68).

Ideal Supplementary Nutrient Intake for Hormonal Health

Nutrient	For Maintenance	For Correction	For Extra Bone-Building
Vitamins			
Vitamin A	17,500iu	22,500	
as retinol	7500iu		
as beta-carotene	10,000iu	15,000iu	
Vitamin C	1000mg	2000–4000mg	
Vitamin D	400iu		
Vitamin E	150mg (200iu)	500mg (600iu)	
B1 (Thiamine)	25mg		
B2 (Riboflavin)	25mg		
B3 (Niacin)	25mg		
B5 (Pantothenic acid)	25mg		
B6 (Pyridoxine)	25mg	50–100mg	
B12	10mcg	20mcg	
Folic acid	100mcg	400–1000mcg	
Biotin	50mcg		

Minerals

Calcium	350mg	500mg	600mg
Magnesium	200mg	300mg	400mg
Zinc	15mg	20mg	25mg
Iron	10mg		
Manganese	5mg		10mg
Chromium	50mcg	100mcg	
Selenium	100mcg		
Boron	1mg		3mg
Copper			2mg

Beneficial Fats

GLA	150mg	250mg	
EPA (fish oil)	200mg	300mg	
Flax oil (vegans)	1000mg	1500mg (instead of EPA)	

In practical terms, the easiest way to achieve these levels is to supplement:

- A good, all-round multivitamin and multimineral plus extra vitamin C
- Evening primrose oil or borage (starflower) oil for GLA

Plus, for those with special needs:

- extra vitamin E
- either a B complex or individual B6 and folic acid
- a bone mineral complex for extra calcium, magnesium, zinc, etc

Good supplement companies provide preparations that can meet these needs. Take your supplements with food, unless otherwise stated. Many vitamins help to boost your energy levels so they are best taken with breakfast or lunch. Calcium and magnesium have a calming effect and are best taken with dinner, especially if you have difficulty getting to sleep. Most important of all, stick to your supplement program every day. It can take three months before you notice the beneficial effects. They are worth waiting for.

REFERENCES

Part 2

1. "Report of Cancer Incidence and Prevalence Projections," East Anglian Cancer Intelligence Unit, Department of Community Medicine, University of Cambridge, Macmillan Cancer Relief (June 1997)
2. Herman-Giddens Dr M. University of North Carolina. Article in *Daily Mail* by Gaby Hinscliff, medical reporter. Originally published in *Journal of Paediatrics* (9 April 1997)
3. Women's Nutritional Advisory Service, "Social implications of premenstrual syndrome – 11 years on" (1996)
4. Coutinho E. "Progress in management of endometriosis," *Proceedings of the Fourth World Congress on Endometriosis 25–28 May 1994*, Salvador, Bahia, Brazil, Parthenon Publishing Press
5. Carruthers M. *The Male Menopause*, HarperCollins (1996)
6. Cadbury D. *The Feminisation of Nature*, Hamish Hamilton (1997)
7. Colborn T. Myers and Dumanoski, *Our Stolen Future*, Little, Brown (1997).
8. "Annual Report of the Working Party on Pesticide Residues: 1996," MAFF Health and Safety Executive
9. Vom Saal F. "Sexual differentiation in mammals; in chemically induced alterations in sexual and functional development: the wildlife-human connection," T. Colborn and C. Clement (eds), Princetown Scientific Publishing, pp 17–38 (1992)
10. Bergkvist L et al. "The risk of breast cancer after estrogen and estrogen-progestin replacement," *N Engl J Med* 1989; 32: 293–297
11. Colditz G et al. "The use of estrogen and progestins and the risk of breast cancer in postmenopausal women," *N Engl J Med* 1995; 332: 1589–93
12. Rodriguez C et al. "Estrogen replacement therapy and fatal ovarian cancer," *Am J Epidemiology* 1995; 141(9): 828–35
13. Lee J. *Viewpoint Optimum Nutrition*, 1997; 10.1: 12–13

Part 3

1. Grant Dr E. *Sexual Chemistry, Understanding our Hormones, the Pill and HRT* Cedar (1994)
2. Ibid.
3. Barnes B, and Bradley SG. *Planning for a Healthy Baby*, Vemilion, second ed. (1992)

4. *Lancet* (26 July 1980) also in *Good Health Guide,* Bloomsbury Health Publisher

5. Rushton A. "Fertility rites," *Optimum Nutrition,* vol 7, no. 1 (Spring 1994)

6. *Optimum Nutrition,* vol 11, no. 1, p 15 (1998)

7. Wynne M. & Wynne A. *The Case for Preconception Care of Men and Women* AB Academic Publishers (1991)

8. Czeizel et al. *N Engl J Med* 1992; 327

9. Wachstein M. and Graffeo L. "Influence of vitamin B6 on the incidence of preclampsia." *Obstet Gyn* 1956; 8: 177

10. Baurdon F. "HRT: The Myth is Exploded," *What Doctors Don't Tell You,* vol 4, no. 9

11. Aura M. et al. "Medroxyprogesterone interferes with ovarian steroid protection against coronary vaso spasm," *Nature Medicine* 1997; 3(3)

12. *N Engl J Med* (1993)

13. Bawdon F. (See Note 10 above).

14. Lee J. "Osteoporosis reversal with transdermal progesterone," *The Lancet,* 1990; 336: 1327

15. "Milk Increases Osteoporosis Risk," *Optimum Nutrition,* vol 11, no. 1, p 15 (1998)

16. Neil, Kate, "Osteoporosis" *Optimum Nutrition,* vol 9, no. 1 (1996)

17. "A Significant Advance in Bone Disease Management," Metra Biosystems Inc. (1994)

18. Lee J. with Virginia Hopkins, *What Your Doctor May Not Tell You About Menopause* Warner Books (1996)

19. Ibid.

20. Sellman S. "Tamoxifen – A major medical mistake?" *Nexus* June–July 1998

21. Grant Dr E. *Sexual Chemistry, Understanding our Hormones, the Pill and HRT* Cedar (1994)

22. *British Journal of Cancer* 1996; 73: 1552–1555

23. London R. Bloomsbury Health Publisher.

24. *Food, Nutrition and the Prevention of Cancer: A Global Perspective* World Cancer Research Fund/American Institute for Cancer Research (1997)

25. Ibid.

26. *Good Health Guide* Bloomsbury Health Publisher (1987)

27. Vessey M. et al. "Epidemiology of endometriosis in women attending family planning clinics," *BMJ* 1993; 306: 182–4

28. Mills D. "Endometriosis Epidemic," *Optimum Nutrition*, vol 8, no. 2 (1995)

29. Whitehead N. et al. "Megaloblastic changes in the cervical epithelium. Association with oral contraceptive therapy and reversal with folic acid," *JAMA* 1973; 226: 1421–4

30. Rodriguez et al. "Oestrogen replacement therapy and fatal ovarian cancer," *Am J Epidemiology* 1995; 141(9)

Part 4

1. "Oestrogen and Progesterone Explained," *Nutrition Bites*, Issue 3, *Female Hormone Imbalance Syndromes*, Lamberts (1997)

2. Ibid.

3. Ibid.

4. Carpenter L. "Heard the one about the Pill? It's a killer!" in Neil K. *Balancing Hormones Naturally*, ION Press (1994)

5. Kuhnz et al. *Influences of high doses of vitamin C on the bio availability and the serum protein binding of levonorgestrel in women using a combination oral contraceptive*, Elsevier Science Inc., New York, USA (1995)

6. Grant Dr E. (see Note 1, Part 3 above)

7. Bawdon F. (see Note 10, Part 3 above)

8. McTaggart L. "HRT: More Bad News," *What Doctors Don't Tell You*, vol 4, no. 10

9. "Immunomodulation of the Mother during Pregnancy," *Medical Hypotheses*, Institute for Research and Reproduction, Parel, Bombay, India 1991; 35(2): 159–164

Part 5

1. Messina M and Messina V. "Increasing use of soyfoods and their potential role in cancer prevention," *Perspectives in Practice* 1991; 91(7): 836–40

2. Dwyer J et al. "Tofu and soy drinks contain phytoestrogens," *J Am Diet Assoc* 1994; 94(7): 739–43

3. Beckman N. "Phytoestrogens and compounds that affect estrogen metabolism – part 2," *Aust J Med Herbalism* 1995; 7(2): 27–33

4. Dittmar F. et al. "Premenstrual syndrome: treatment with a phytopharmaceutical," *TW Gynakol*, 1992; 5(1): 60–68

5. Mills S. *Out of the Earth* Viking, Penguin, London (1991)

INDEX

RELATED BOOKS BY THE CROSSING PRESS

Healing Yourself Naturally

By Judy Jacka

This book gives a clear explanation of the natural way to deal with illness and disease. Judy Jacka's book rests on the holistic view that the body can balance itself.

$18.95 • Paper • ISBN 0-89594-954-7

Good Food: The Comprehensive Food & Nutrition Resource

By Margaret M. Wittenberg

An exceptionally well-organized, up-to-date, and easily accessible treatise on food and nutrition. Wittenberg delineates a direct connection between food and quality of life.
—Susan Jane Cheney, Food Writer/Columnist

$18.95 • Paper • ISBN 0-89594-746-3

The Optimum Nutrition Bible

By Patrick Holford

Optimum nutrition means giving yourself the best possible intake of nutrients to allow your body to be as healthy as possible. This book shows you precisely how to achieve this, and gives a step-by-step plan to create your own personal supplement program.

$16.95 • Paper • ISBN 1-58091-015-7

Perimenopause

By Bernard Cortese, M.D.

This book describes the changes that may take place, discusses the pros and cons of hormone replacement therapy (HRT), offers alternative treatments, and stresses the importance of exercise, proper diet, and stress management.

$11.95 • Paper • ISBN 0-89594-914-8

Rejuvenate: A 21-Day Natural Detox Plan for Optimal Health

By Helene Silver

Rejuvenate gives step-by-step instructions on how to cleanse your body of toxins and rejuvenate both body and mind.

$16.95 • Paper • ISBN 0-89594-938-5

Vitamins, Minerals & Supplements

By Gayle Skowronski and Beth Petro Roybal

Vitamins, Minerals & Supplements gives general information about the role of supplements in nutrition and how to choose them wisely.

$11.95 • Paper • ISBN 0-89594-935-0

To receive a current catalog from The Crossing Press
please call toll-free, 800-777-1048.
Visit our Web site: www.crossingpress.com